EDUCATION GROUPS FOR MEN WHO BATTER

The Duluth Model

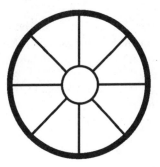

Ellen Pence
Michael Paymar

With Contributions by:
Tineke Ritmeester
Melanie Shepard

 SPRINGER **P**UBLISHING **C**OMPANY • **N**EW **Y**ORK

Springer Publishing Company, Inc.
536 Broadway
New York, NY 10012

94 95 96 97 / 5 4 3 2

Library of Congress Cataloging-in-Publication Data

Pence, Ellen.
    Education groups for men who batter : the Duluth model / Ellen Pence, Michael Paymar.
        p.   cm.
    Includes bibliographical references and index.
    ISBN 0–8291–7990–8
    1. Abusive men––Counseling of.   2. Abusive men––Rehabilitation.
3. Group relations training.   I. Paymar, Michael.   II. Title.
HV6626.P45   1993
362.82'92––dc20

92–35954
CIP

Printed in the United States of America

EDUCATION GROUPS FOR MEN WHO BATTER

The Duluth Model

Dr. Kathy McCloskey
University of Hartford
Graduate Institute of Professional Psychology
103 Woodland St.
Hartford, CT 06105

Ellen Pence is one of the original organizers of the Duluth Domestic Abuse Intervention Project. She has worked within the battered women's movement at local, state, and national levels since 1975. As an international lecturer, author, and producer of several training videos on community responses to battering, she has influenced much of the thinking in the criminal justice system on this issue. Ms. Pence is currently a graduate student at the Ontario Institute of Education in Toronto.

Michael Paymar, a licensed social worker, has worked with men who batter in jails and in educational groups since 1981. He is currently the coordinator at the National Training Project of the Duluth Domestic Abuse Intervention Project. He has produced several training videos and accompanying manuals for police, court personnel, and facilitators of men's groups. Mr. Paymar, who holds a BA degree in Education from the College of St. Scholastica in Duluth, Minnesota, served eight years on the Duluth City Council. He has lectured extensively throughout North America.

Dedicated to the more than 6000 women
who have sought safety and protection
in the Duluth shelter
and to those who have worked
to provide that protection

Contents

CONTRIBUTORS

Tineke Ritmeester, PhD, is a Dutch feminist, scholar, and activist. She holds an MA in German Area Studies and a PhD in German Literature, both from Washington University in St. Louis. She has been active in the battered women's movement since 1979, and was cofounder of the first autonomous women's shelter in Tuviegen, Germany. She currently teaches Women's Studies and International Studies at the University of Minnesota, Duluth. She is a member of the Modern Language Association, the National Organization for Women, and the National Women's Studies Association.

Melanie Shepard, PhD, is an associate professor in the Department of Social Work at the University of Minnesota, Duluth. Dr. Shepard has provided research consultation for the Duluth Domestic Abuse Intervention Project since 1984 and has facilitated groups for both men and women. She received her MSSW from the University of Wisconsin, Madison, and her PhD from the University of Minnesota.

ACKNOWLEDGMENTS

This curriculum was developed with the help of dozens of people who have been involved in the Duluth Domestic Abuse Intervention Project (DAIP) over the past 12 years. Although women active in the shelter movement provided the leadership for this project, practitioners in many agencies have helped shape what it is today.

Dr. Anne Ganley provided the shelter staff, probation officers, DAIP staff, and counselors with the initial training on a counseling model for court-mandated abusers. Throughout the 12 years of the project she has continued to offer advice and support. She has provided valuable input in her critique of this curriculum in its various stages of development.

We recognize the dozens of battered women who came to educational groups organized by the Duluth shelter, viewed our films, critiqued our definitions, added topics, deleted topics, and provided us with the understanding needed to make the training tapes. They have made a valuable contribution to this work

We must also not overlook the men in the Duluth program who have endured 8 years of the project testing these ideas. Throughout this book are excerpts from more than 100 taped group sessions.

The Minnesota Coalition for Battered Women and its more than 50 member programs have, during the past 14 years, worked to create a body of law that gives each community in this state the tools needed to protect women who turn to the police and courts for help. The Duluth program would be an impossibility without their work.

Special thanks go to Kate Regan, who spent many hours editing the constant flow of drafts, and to Coral McDonnell and Nancy Helgeson, who typed and retyped our manuscript.

This book is a description of the collective work of these many individuals.

INTRODUCTION

In 1980 in Duluth, Minnesota, after a particularly brutal "domestic" homicide, the Duluth Domestic Abuse Intervention Project (DAIP) found a relatively receptive community willing to experiment with new practices to confront the problem of men's violence toward their partners. Organizers from DAIP debated, cajoled, and negotiated with law enforcement agencies, the justice system, and human service providers to go beyond a superficial examination of the flaws in the system to committing to a comprehensive overhaul of the police, court, and human service systems' response to these cases. The project argued for practices that would hold offenders accountable and place the onus of intervention on the community, not on the individual woman being beaten. Ensuring women's safety would be the community's responsibility. Within a year policies and procedures were developed and a community experiment began.

With a dramatic increase in arrests and prosecution, the city of Duluth had to contend with another major problem: What to do with all of these men? Unless there were aggravating circumstances, the courts refused to impose jail sentences on first offenders without first giving them an opportunity to rehabilitate themselves.

We asked a small group of activists in the battered women's movement to come to Duluth and critique an educational curriculum that we had developed as a guide for counselors to use in court-mandated groups. Barbara Hart and Susan Schechter from the Women's Leadership Institute, and Joe Morse and Miguel Gil from EMERGE in Boston spent several days of intense discussion with us. Our initial draft of a curriculum seemed to be philosophically adrift. Barbara, Susan, Joe, and Miguel guided us by asking questions from the standpoint of women who are battered. Why is she the target of his violence? How does his violence impact the balance of power in their relationship? What did he think could change by hitting her? Why does he assume he is entitled to have power in the relationship? How does the community support his use of violence against her? These questions and continued dialogue helped to shape our analysis—of and ultimately our approach to—working with batterers.

The DAIP has worked with thousands of men over the years. As a monitor of the justice system, we pressure that system to impose consequences for continued acts of violence. As an organization committed to social change, we challenge local institutions to think about their own complicity through their actions or inactions. As an organization that works directly with offenders, we confront batterers' behavior and question their beliefs in the most compassionate way we can.

This book describes a major component of what has become known as the "Duluth Model." It explains the methods used in our work with men who batter and offers group process techniques for facilitators of men's groups. It is our hope that this book will assist in the understanding of the complex nature of battering and of the man who batters—his thinking, the intent of his actions, and the impact of his violent behavior on the woman he batters, on his children, and ultimately on himself.

We must never forget the danger a woman faces living with a batterer or attempting to leave him. We have no illusions that most men will stop their violence and give up their power, but we have an unshakable belief that within us all is the capacity to change.

Chapter 1

Theoretical Framework for Understanding Battering

Education is never neutral.—Paulo Freire

Providing an educational process for men who batter their partners is not a neutral endeavor. Each facilitator conducts a group within a community, a program, and a personal philosophical framework that either supports a man's process of change toward nonviolence or reinforces his dominance over the woman he batters. Each statement, handout, assignment, role play, video, or story used in a group is grounded in a theory.

Theory guides and informs practice. The curriculum described in this book is based on the theory that violence is used to control people's behavior. This curriculum is designed to be used within a community using its institutions to diminish the power of batterers over their victims and to explore with each abusive man the intent and source of his violence and the possibilities for change through seeking a different kind of relationship with women.

Often a fine line separates those of us who teach the class from those court mandated to attend. We've all been socialized in a culture that values power, a culture in which the thinking that we challenge in the groups is present in every aspect of our daily lives. Our schools, churches, and places of work are all structured hierarchically. All of us have engaged in at least some of the tactics batterers use to control their partners. To challenge the norm requires challenging ourselves. In many ways using theories that ignore intent and focusing instead on violence as the result of stress or anger or an inability to express

1

feelings would be easier than what this curriculum offers. It would be more palatable not only to the men but also to those of us who teach the classes. But in the end it is less honest because it fails to acknowledge the real experiences of women who live with men who batter.

In 1984, based on group interviews with women attending educational classes offered by the Duluth battered women's shelter, we began developing a framework for describing the behavior of men who physically and emotionally abuse their partners. Many of the women criticized theories that described battering as cyclical rather than as a constant force in their relationship; that attributed the violence to men's inability to cope with stress; and that failed to acknowledge fully the intention of batterers to gain control over their partners' actions, thoughts, and feelings. Challenging the assumptions about why women stay with men who beat them, more than 200 battered women in Duluth who participated in 30 educational sessions sponsored by the shelter designed the Power and Control Wheel (see Figure 1.1 and Appendix 1), which depicts the primary abusive behaviors experienced by women living with men who batter. It illustrates that violence is part of a pattern of behaviors rather than isolated incidents of abuse or cyclical explosions of pent-up anger, frustration, or painful feelings. (Appendix 1 is a larger version of the Power and Control Wheel for photocopying.)

A batterer's use of physical assaults or sexual abuse is often infrequent, but it reinforces the power of the other tactics on the wheel (e.g., emotional abuse, isolation, threats of taking the children) that are used at random and eventually undermine his partner's ability to act autonomously.

Although many men experience themselves as out of control or controlled by emotional outbursts when battering, their behaviors are not without intent. They may become almost automatic, but with few exceptions each abusive act can be traced to the intent of the batterer. For example, a man may use degrading names, calling his partner a whore or slut before grabbing, shaking, or slapping her. Although he does not think, "First I'm going to objectify her, then I'm going to hit her," objectifying his partner through degrading names allows him to hit the object he has created rather than his partner. This pattern may be so ingrained in his history and cultural experience that it seems second nature to him.

The tactics used by batterers reflect the tactics used by many groups or individuals in positions of power. Each of the tactics depicted on the Power and Control Wheel are typical of behaviors used by groups of people who dominate others. They are the tactics employed to sustain racism, ageism, classism, heterosexism, anti-Semitism, and many other forms of group domination. Men in particular are taught these tactics in both their families of origin and through their experiences in a culture that teaches men to dominate.

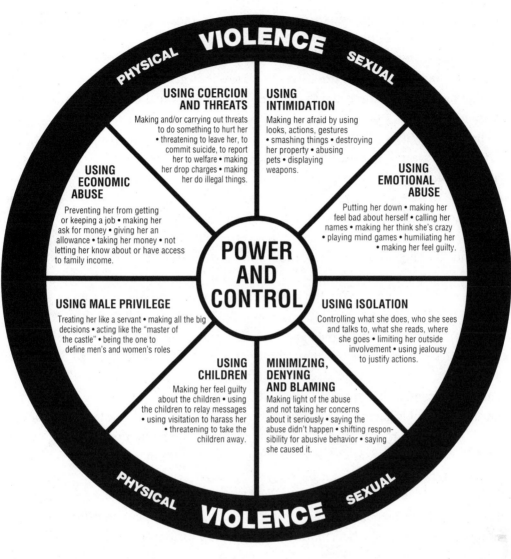

Figure 1.1   Power and Control Wheel.

Batterers, like those who intervene to help them, have been immersed in a culture that supports relationships of dominance. This cultural acceptance of dominance is rooted in the assumption that, based on differences, some people have the legitimate right to master others. Southern whites proclaimed segregation to be God's plan carried out in the interest of "less developed" Southern blacks. Through their institutions, European Americans have for the last five centuries dominated Native American people. When the military failed to completely annihilate them, the churches and, most recently, social service agencies were called on to assimilate them, as if making indigenous people "European" would elevate rather than diminish them as a people.

Those in control use societal institutions to justify, support, and enforce the relationship of dominance and make extensive efforts to obtain general acceptance of the premises that hierarchy is natural and that those at the bottom are there because of their own deficiencies.

The consciousness of separateness prevails. Differences among people are not celebrated and treasured but used as a reason to dominate. When relationships of dominance become the norm in a culture, then all individuals within it are socialized to internalize those values or exist on the fringe of society. Individuals mirror global and national relationships in their own interpersonal relationships.

Most batterers are informed by cultural messages justifying dominance and vigorously defend their beliefs as absolute truths with slogans such as "Someone has to be in charge," "You can't have two captains for one ship," "If I don't control my child/wife/partner, she will control me," "God made man first, which means he is supposed to rule woman," or "This is my child, it is my responsibility to control him."

The consciousness of both men and women in this society is shaped by their experiences of this system and all of the forces that work within it. Yet not all men batter women even though all men have been socialized in a society that grants them certain gender privileges. Not all parents physically punish their children even though all parents in this country have the legal right to do so. Likewise, not all white people commit violent acts of racism, yet all whites have been exposed to powerful socializing experiences that tell them they are superior to people of color. Ultimately we must each be accountable for the choices we make.

The history of a man who batters is often a history of childhood abuse; exposure to male role models who have shown hostile attitudes toward women; exposure to women-hating environments; alcoholism; racial and class oppression; and the denial of love and nurturing as a child. Clearly many men who we work with need to find ways to heal from the sexual and physical abuse they experienced as children. We can't discount their pain and their scars. Nevertheless, these individual experiences can easily become both an explanation of why a man batters and an excuse to continue his violence. To change long-held patterns, men must acknowledge the destructive nature of their present behaviors and accept the responsibility for their actions. They are not, however, responsible for creating the many forces that have shaped their thinking. Although the men are not victims of sexism as are the women they beat, they are dehumanized by their socialization.

Not all batterers are the same. A few are mentally ill, some have no apparent remorse for their violence, and some, if not morally motivated to change, are at least miserable enough to want their situation to be different. Still others are truly appalled at their own behavior. The rationalizations of abusers for their behaviors, like those of other individuals and groups who dominate through force, often result in the abusers not only portraying but, in some sense, believing themselves to be the victims of those they beat. This delusion is often reinforced by the practices of police, judges, social workers, clergy, educators, therapists, reporters, and other representatives of society's institutions.

Abusers are capable of personal transformation, and many of them will make extensive changes if certain conditions exist. First, the abuser must be held fully accountable for his use of violence by a community that establishes and enforces consequences for continued acts of abuse. Second, he must have an environment that is nonviolent, nonjudgmental, and respectful of women and children in which to start making those changes. And finally, he must be willing to work through a long process during which he is painfully honest with himself and becomes accountable to the woman he has harmed.

THE ISSUE OF GENDER

Throughout this curriculum we use male pronouns to refer to batterers and female pronouns to refer to those who are battered. Dealing with gay and lesbian battering is beyond the scope of this book. We use gender-specific terms not only because the curriculum is for men who batter, but because battering is not a gender-neutral issue.

In intimate heterosexual relationships where violence is occurring, the primary aggressors are typically men, and the victims are women. Every source of data, from police reports to hospital emergency rooms, from counseling centers to divorce courts, points to an enormous gender disparity in who is initiating the violence, who is more physically harmed, and who is seeking safety from the violence.

Ty

Sometimes I would really push her to hit me or to brush up against me and then I would really feel justified in hitting her. I'd just think she hit me first.

Violence in the family is directly linked to status in the family and to socialization. Men are culturally prepared for their role of master of the home even though they must often physically enforce the "right" to exercise this role. They are socialized to be dominant and women to be subordinate.

This doesn't mean that women never use violence. A person who is kicked or punched or spit on or cursed or dragged from room to room or thrown down on the floor usually responds with some kind of physical defense. Women often kick, scratch, and bite the men who beat them, but that does not constitute mutual battering.

Mutual battering occurs when both parties engage in a series of abusive and controlling behaviors, coupled with the threat or use of violence to control what the other partner thinks, does, or feels.

Women's violence toward their male partners that is neither in self-defense nor in response to being battered is rare but can still be very dangerous. During the past 10 years the DAIP has worked with just under 100 women who have physically assaulted their partners (this represents 3.5 % of offenders mandated to DAIP). In seven of these cases, the men were unable to leave the situation without increasing their partner's violence. These seven men, like the thousands of women who have sought safety at the shelter, were being pursued and terrorized by their partners. They, like many battered women, needed legal protection, safe housing, and tremendous emotional support.

What separated those seven men from the 90 other male assault victims was their fear and their inability to leave without their abusers escalating the violence and threats. Most men who live with women who are violent are abusing the women who have assaulted them and can end the violence against them by stopping their own violence or leaving the relationship.

The factors differentiating the enormous social problem of men's violence against women from the violence of women against men are the number of cases and the severity and pattern of the violence used against the victims. The civil protection order and the criminal court process are effective tools for protecting almost all male victims because women rarely engage in "separation violence," the violence that occurs and escalates as victims attempt to leave their abusers. A report issued by the Minnesota Coalition for Battered Women on January 28, 1991, documented the murders of 27 Minnesota women who were killed in 1990 by their male partners; half of them were trying to leave their relationships. None of the public documents indicates that any of the men killed by their partners during the same year were attempting to leave the relationship.

BLAMING OF WOMEN FOR MEN'S VIOLENCE

The use of the tactics on the Power and Control Wheel result in men's domination of women physically, sexually, emotionally, and spiritually. When a woman is repeatedly battered, she experiences severe physical, psychological, and spiritual trauma. When she manifests the effects of these attacks or fights back she is labeled by the batterer, and by the system that colludes with him, as defective. She is described by him as a provocative bitch, a whore, a junkie, a bad mother, a violent drunk, a liar, a manhater, a thief, and a woman out to get him. She is labeled by the community as an enabler, a reluctant witness, a codependent partner, a woman caught in a honeymoon phase, a nonassertive woman suffering from learned helplessness, a mother with poor parenting skills, a drug or alcohol abuser, a violent person, and a self-destructive woman. Like any person or group at the bottom of an abusive hierarchical order, she is thought to be there because something is wrong with her. He defines her this way, and the system backs him up.

She is studied in her postvictimized state and is judged to be lacking. She is compared with "nonbattered" women in study after study, and the difference between the two is defined as the cause of her problem. The question of why this woman is the one who gets hit is answered by theories of academics and professionals that sound suspiciously like the claims of her batterer. She lacks certain skills and attitudes, and her behavior is not quite right. He is reinforced; she is revictimized. He becomes a more cooperative client; she becomes more problematic.

Battered women, like nonbattered women, come from all backgrounds and act in many different ways. Some battered women are incredibly kind and loving; others are not. Some never touch alcohol; some are heavy drinkers. Some are monogamous; others are not. But rarely can a person get involved in this issue and stay clear about how irrelevant all of that is. Our system and those of us who are its agents search for an answer to the question: Is she an innocent victim, or did she somehow play a part in her victimization? How we answer that question dictates how we respond to him as a perpetrator and to her as a victim.

The Duluth model of interagency intervention and the groups for men are structured to keep all of us—the men, the group leaders, and those in the court system—from engaging in victim-blaming practices.

COMMON BELIEFS OF BATTERERS

The 26-week curriculum described in this book is designed to help men change from using the behaviors on the Power and Control Wheel, which result in authoritarian and destructive relationships, to using the behaviors on the Equality Wheel (see Figure 1.2 and Appendix 2),which form the basis for egalitarian relationships. (Appendix 2 is a larger version of the Equality Wheel for photocopying.)

Although men in groups may stop using violence, eliminating other behaviors on the Power and Control Wheel is a much longer process. If a batterer does not have a personal commitment to give up his position of power, he will eventually return to the use of threats or violence to gain control. Long-term change and a true commitment to egalitarian relationships necessitates a long, honest look at deeply held beliefs, a resolve to handle conflict differently, and an honest examination of why he wants a woman in his life. His change process requires practicing the things we can teach him with the hope that those alternative behaviors become his new norm. Every aspect of the Duluth

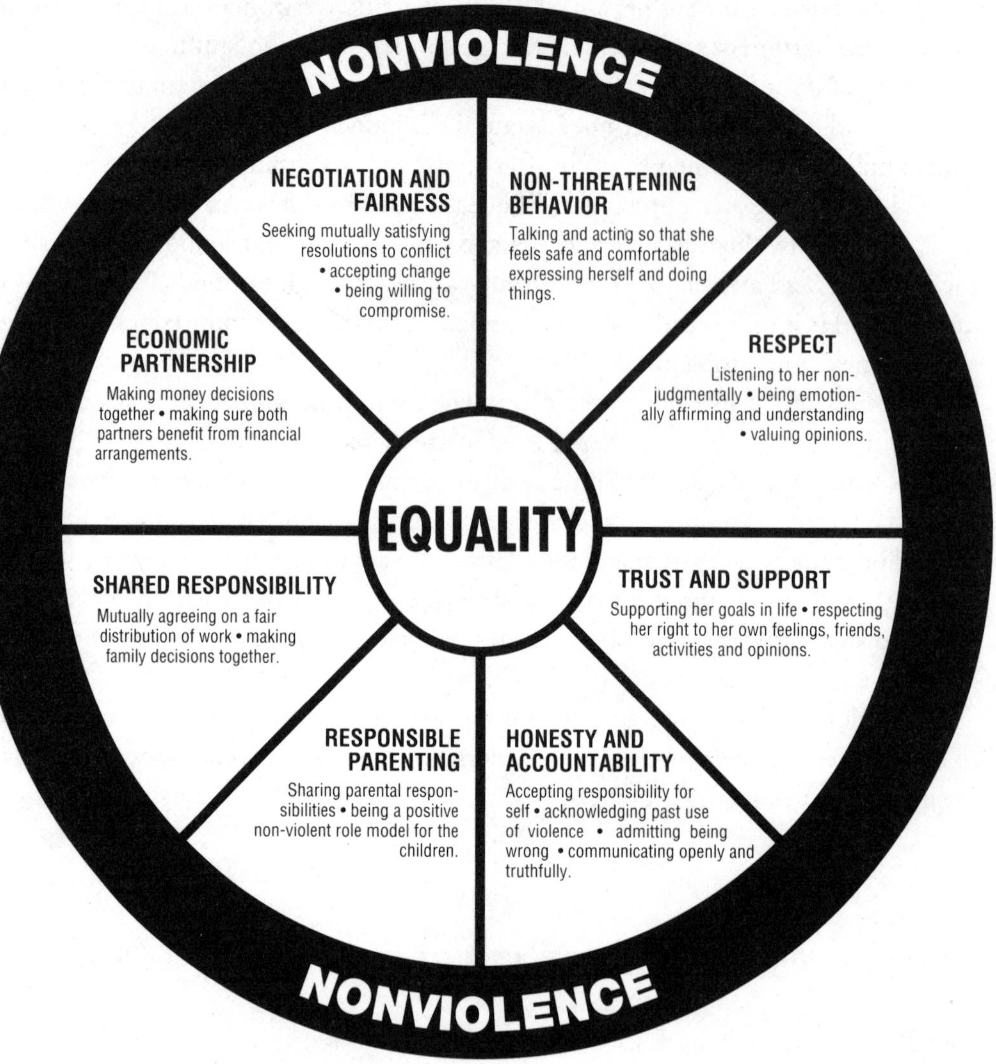

NONVIOLENCE

NEGOTIATION AND FAIRNESS
Seeking mutually satisfying resolutions to conflict • accepting change • being willing to compromise.

NON-THREATENING BEHAVIOR
Talking and acting so that she feels safe and comfortable expressing herself and doing things.

ECONOMIC PARTNERSHIP
Making money decisions together • making sure both partners benefit from financial arrangements.

RESPECT
Listening to her non-judgmentally • being emotionally affirming and understanding • valuing opinions.

EQUALITY

SHARED RESPONSIBILITY
Mutually agreeing on a fair distribution of work • making family decisions together.

TRUST AND SUPPORT
Supporting her goals in life • respecting her right to her own feelings, friends, activities and opinions.

RESPONSIBLE PARENTING
Sharing parental responsibilities • being a positive non-violent role model for the children.

HONESTY AND ACCOUNTABILITY
Accepting responsibility for self • acknowledging past use of violence • admitting being wrong • communicating openly and truthfully.

NONVIOLENCE

Figure 1.2   Equality Wheel.

intervention process and the curriculum is designed to challenge a lifelong pattern of thinking, rationalizing, and acting that leads to violence and other forms of abuse.

A man's thinking and view of the world reflect his beliefs. Throughout countless discussions during the 26 weeks, belief statements will emerge. There are many structured exercises in this curriculum to assist men in understanding the origins and implications of their beliefs.

In writing this curriculum we met with five women who have been battered and with four men who have completed the educational program and remained nonviolent for a year or longer. Many of their comments have been included in this section. We asked them which beliefs frequently articulated by batterers would be most important to discuss in groups, and from their responses compiled the following list.

1. Anger causes violence.

> or

- If I get angry enough, I will blow and become violent.

Bob

I look back now and I see that I was always angry. That got me places. It made her watch out, it made it so I didn't have to do much around the house. She didn't dare ask me to. It kept the kids from hassling me. I'd always be angry and as soon as she'd do something I didn't like, come home late or put the dishes away too noisily, then I'd jump up and break something or slam something, and sometimes I'd hit her. Then I'd say she got me angry and that's why I hit her.

I think in a lot of ways I used my anger to constantly intimidate her. After she got the protection order against me, I moved out and didn't see her for a month. Then we got back together. I kept thinking, "I can't get mad, don't blow it, keep cool." I thought the problem was just my getting mad. After a while it started making sense to me that I couldn't spend the rest of my life hoping I didn't get mad. I had to start thinking about why I was mad all the time.

2. Women are manipulative.

Jack

I knew that my wife was taking money, $3 here, $4 there. Every time she'd go grocery shopping or do anything, she always wanted me to give her cash. I started suspecting that she was storing it away.

One day, we got into a fight about something and I hit her. Then I started yelling at her to tell me where the money was. She said she didn't have any money. Well, I just let it go. Later on I found out that she did have about $80 stashed away that she planned on using to leave me.

When I found out about the money, I brought it up in the men's group, and I said she had stolen the money from me and lied about it. Next thing I know, I'm the one on the hot seat. What I came to see is that what I saw as lying was, from her point of view, survival in the situation. I remember that group. It sticks out in my mind. We discussed ways that we had acted when we thought a situation was unfair at work or with friends. A lot of the guys talked about being in the service. I know now the things I thought of as lying and cheating were partly her way of trying to live with me.

3. Women think of men as paychecks.

Pete

I didn't think she'd ever leave me because I knew she had no education and no work experience. I pretty much thought she'd never walk out the door.

When we talked about "men as paychecks to women" in the group, I was sitting in the group thinking that's true and that's the way I want to keep it. I knew that was why she was still with me. I said it wasn't fair and I didn't like the fact that I was thought of as a paycheck, but in the back of my mind I knew, or thought, that as long as this was true, she wouldn't leave.

About six months into the group she left me. I remember thinking that I'd get her back just because she couldn't make it out there alone. She did, she made it without me.

I realize now that being a paycheck to her was a bad thing for me. Now I know a lot of what we talked about in group was true even though I wasn't sincere about the things I was saying. I don't think you realize what you could lose, what you're giving up, until she actually leaves you.

4. If a man is hurt, it's OK or natural for him to hurt back.

Bob

When we watched the videotapes in group, most of the discussions would be from the lady's point of view.

Well, one day I was in there pitching for the guy and Paul, the group leader, says, "Bob, you've got a kind word to say for all of these guys. That's good, but I'm starting to think there's something behind all these kind words that you should talk about." Finally, I just said, "I'm never going to let someone hurt me without hurting him back." That goes way back to being a kid and not being able to protect myself.

The whole group ended up talking a lot about how we protected ourselves as kids. One guy's dad beat the shit out of him every day, and he had that same thing in him about he'd never let it happen again. Anyway it's funny how you do things at one point in your life that help you and later on, you're still doing them not so much because you need to but because you still feel like you need to. I got a lot out of that group. It made me start relaxing about this "eye-for-an-eye" attitude.

5. Smashing things isn't abusive, it's venting.

The idea that punching walls, throwing and breaking objects, or slamming doors is a healthy release of anger continually surfaces in men's groups. Challenging the nature of this behavior typically brings the response, "At least I didn't hit her." Facilitators can discuss how a man's past use of violence makes such outbursts even more intimidating.

Sam

After I got arrested, that was my biggest defense. I'd smash the wall, knock shit over, and just look at her and say, "I didn't hit you, did I?"

6. **Women's libbers hate men.**

> or

- The shelter wants marriages to break up.

When a group of 15 abusive men, all required by the court to participate in the program, claims that shelters break up marriages, denial is running rampant. Nevertheless, it's easy for facilitators to get drawn into this discussion.

Sally

At first I didn't want to go to the women's groups, but Terry was always saying I was the one who needed groups. I started going and after a while I really liked them. Then Terry got this thing in his head about how they were all lesbians at the shelter. He, of course, had different ways of calling them that.

One day he came home from group and told me this story about how a guy's wife was locked in a room at the shelter until she agreed to sign divorce papers. The guy was suing the shelter. If he ever wanted to make a point that I would argue with, he'd say, "Bob says" or "Carol says" (his group leaders), but if I brought up something somebody at the shelter said, he'd say, "What the hell do they know? They just make their money off divorces."

I know that nothing was more threatening to him than the shelter people because to him, they were symbols of women who didn't need men. He wanted me to need him, he just would never believe that I wanted to be with him. Eventually I didn't.

7. **Women want to be dominated by men.**

> or

- If women didn't like it, they wouldn't stay.

> or

- Some women are masochistic.

> or

- Women ask for it.

This is the ultimate Catch-22 for women. Women have been taught from the cradle how to survive in a world where men hold most of the power. These survival techniques include deferring to men, influencing men to make things happen, and attaching themselves to men who can provide for and protect them. These behaviors and the corresponding consciousness they create are then turned against women in the form of labels: "masochistic," "codependent," or "addicted to men."

Men learn at an early age that male dominance is somehow "natural." Decades of television programs reflecting the views of mainstream America have perpetuated this concept. It is reinforced in the privacy of a young boy's bedroom as he takes his first look at pornography. There is the submitting woman, offering free access, wanting to be dominated and hurt by a man. As he looks at her, he pictures himself as the dominator.

8.   Men batter women because they are insecure.

FACILITATOR: Why do you think the man in the film was questioning his wife about what she had been doing all day?

JIM: He was insecure.

FACILITATOR: How do you mean insecure? What does that mean to you?

JIM: Insecure means when you're feeling out of control.

FACILITATOR: Is that how you define insecure—out of control?

JIM: Yeah, sort of not knowing what you're doing.

FACILITATOR: Okay, let's define insecure before we go on. Anybody else have a definition for insecure?

MARK: Insecure is when you have an idea of how things are supposed to happen and then it doesn't happen that way.

FACILITATOR: So does that mean if your kid doesn't go to bed when you think she should that you'll end up feeling insecure?

MARK: Only if you can't get her to go to bed on time or if it's a baby and you can't get her to quit crying, then you feel like you can't make things happen the way they're supposed to.

FACILITATOR: Any additions to this? OK, so the guy in the film comes home at 5 and his wife is gone and she came home at 6. Now he's insecure because he thinks she should be home when he gets home—is that what you meant, Jim?

JIM: Yeah, he's supposed to go to work and she's supposed to be there when he gets home.

FACILITATOR: Who gets to decide how things are supposed to be? For example, in the film, do you think the woman thinks she is supposed to be home at 5?

JIM: Yeah, she knows the rules.

FACILITATOR: How many men here want your partner to be home when you get home? (Four men raise their hands.)

FACILITATOR: Why?

JACK: 'Cause that's when it's time to eat and for the family to be together.

FACILITATOR: So if she isn't home when you get home, are you insecure?

JACK: It depends.

FACILITATOR: On what?

JACK: On if she's been doing it a lot, where she is, if I know where she is. It depends on a lot of things.

FACILITATOR: Do you think the guy in the film was feeling insecure?

JACK: Yeah, because she was out with Sara, not because it was dinnertime. I think he thinks that if his wife runs with this Sara, she'll start getting ideas.

FACILITATOR: What ideas will she get? What do you think, Jim?

JIM: Yeah, he was insecure because she was out with Sara.

FACILITATOR: For those of you who said you want your partners home when you get home, how did that rule get set? Was it something that both of you agreed on?

JACK: It's not something we both sat down and wrote out, but she expects me home after work too, so it's not just my rule if that's what you're getting at.

FACILITATOR: No, what I'm trying to get at is this idea of security being linked up with having things go the way they are supposed to go. So I'm asking, who decides how things are supposed to go? It seems to me that if I lived by your definition of security, I'd be a basket case because at least twice a day things don't go the way I think they're supposed to go. OK? So back to the film. What was it about her being out with Sara that made him insecure—remembering our definition is that we get insecure when we can't get things to go the way we think they should go.

MARK: He's insecure because she's going to be out with Sara, and he doesn't know what they'll be doing or talking about.

FACILITATOR: He's insecure if he can't control or know what she's doing or talking about?

MARK: Yeah.

FACILITATOR: So he must believe he has the right to control what she does and who she talks to—is that right?

MARK: Yeah, this guy does.

FACILITATOR: What about you, Mark, have you ever interrogated Sue when she's been out?

MARK: Yeah.

FACILITATOR: Do you think you have the right to control what she does and what she thinks?

MARK: I have the right to be concerned if it'll hurt our relationship.

9. A man has the right to choose his partner's friends or associates.

Will (Facilitator)

One day in group, one of the men was talking about how he hated it whenever his partner went to her mother's because her mother hated him and influenced her. So I started asking him a lot of questions trying to get him to see that he didn't have any right to control who his partner talked to. As I was talking, it hit me that I was doing the same thing with my wife. She's been going back to school, and she started volunteering at the women's center. I kept pretending I was supportive, but I'd put out these comments about how she really had to focus on her studies if she wanted to make it. I realized this guy and I were both afraid of the same thing. If she got to be a separate person, she might not still want to be with me.

10. A man can't change if the woman won't.

or

- It takes two to tango.

or

- The woman is half the problem.

Jack

I must have told her a million times that we both had to change to make things work. I still think that's partly true. Both people have to work on a relationship, but it was like I was trading something. I'll quit doing all those things on that chart (pointing to the Control Wheel on the wall) if you'll do this or that. The big wheeler dealer.

Pete

I think just stopping half that crap improves the relationship. It's like you know everything you're doing is screwed up but you keep on, and then in the end you turn to her and say we both have to change. I know my wife has a lot of her own problems; sometimes she's really hard to live with and she does a lot of her own controlling things, but in the end you have to pretty much stick with yourself if you're really going to be different. I know that none of that stuff (his abuse) ever helped the relationship.

Other belief statements commonly articulated include the following:

- Women are just as violent as men.
- Hitting your partner has nothing to do with what kind of parent a man is.
- Sometimes there are no alternatives to violence.
- Somebody has to be in charge.
- Men are naturally jealous.

CREATION OF CONTRADICTION

For many men beliefs are more than a collection of ideas and opinions. They are truisms. The truth is equated with rightness, rightness with something to defend or to preserve. Challenging a long-held belief as being neither the truth nor right but a culturally constructed justification to exploit others will cause varying degrees of defensiveness.

Austin (Facilitator)

I think it was only about the third group I'd done. A guy named Lanny was arguing with everybody about his 13 year-old daughter. He had hit her when she refused to take off her makeup before going out one night. He defended his absolute right as a father to physically force his daughter to take it off. The other guys in the group just didn't support him. After a while we all started talking about the fact that parents don't really own their kids. I had a tape in my car of a Bob Marley song, "Kids come through you, they are of you, but not yours," something like that. So I went out to my car at the break and then played it when we got back together. The discussion was very good about ownership and the right to enforce your "property rights" with violence. Lanny hadn't said anything for quite a while and then all of a sudden he got up and just walked out of the room mumbling, "This just isn't right. There's something drastically wrong here. This is really wrong. . . ."

When we talk about creating contradictions so people have choices, I always think of Lanny. He mumbled all the way to his car. It's one thing when I disagreed with him but when the whole group was disagreeing, it really shook him up.

At the core of the curriculum is the attempt to structure a process by which each man can examine his actions in light of his concept of himself as a man. That examination demands a reflective process that distinguishes between what is in his nature and what is socially constructed. The things that are socially constructed can be changed. Each belief he holds can be traced back to his experiences in his family of origin, his neighborhood, his peer group in school, his military service, his fraternities or other male groups, and to his exposure to the media and its countless images of what it means to be a man. These experiences shape his response to a basic question asked men in the groups over and over again: "Why do you want a woman in your life?"

Many of the men who walk into the group have serious emotional problems. Many men have very poor impulse control; many are insecure, jealous, poor communicators, alcoholic, and drug addicted. Their collective history is filled with violence. These factors are contributors to or modifiers of a man's behavior but they do not cause his violence. They are extensions of his violence and obstacles to meaningful change. The focus must always return to the question of who he is as a man in this world and what that means for a woman in relationship with him.

Chapter 2

The Project Design

In 1981 nine Duluth agencies, under the umbrella of the Domestic Abuse Intervention Project (DAIP), adopted written guidelines, policies, and procedures governing the responses of practitioners in law enforcement, court, and human service agencies to cases of domestic assault. In a city the size of Duluth (population 90,000), city officials estimated that more than 4,000 men were battering, more than 4,000 women were being battered, and more than 8,000 children were watching the abuse.

The Duluth community's decision to use its institutions to intervene in the violence of men against their partners had far-reaching implications.

The participating agencies—the police department, the county jail, the prosecutor's office, the shelter, the county court, the probation department, and three mental health agencies—restricted their employees' use of discretion, and, with the exception of the shelter, opened their records to continuous review by the DAIP,[1] which assumed the role of monitoring agency.

During the first year of organizing this model, participants reached a series of agreements. Most notably, police and court administrators and participating therapists agreed with victim advocates that the act of violence must be made the sole responsibility of the person using it. In other words, the police would no longer base the decision to arrest an assailant on what the victim said or did to contribute to the argument that preceded the assault but would respond based on evidence that an assault had occurred. The jailer would not release a man arrested for domestic assault immediately following booking but would hold him to allow for judicial review of release conditions. The prosecutor would not interpret a woman's request to drop charges as a sign that she was safe but as a probable sign of her vulnerability. The judge would not order a woman to counseling with her abuser to learn how she could communicate with him differently to avoid his beatings. The probation officer would not assume that an assailant is not being violent simply because he has been ordered not to have contact with the woman he was convicted of assaulting. The therapist would not provide marriage counseling to a couple when violence was present. The collective community message to batterers was clear: When you beat your partner, you are not a victim, you are the aggressor. Either stop it or lose increasing amounts of your personal freedom.

Second, the agencies agreed that their contact with batterers was to be a part of a community effort to confront and eliminate their use of violence and not to act as abuser advocates. This agreement is necessary because batterers' counseling programs that are not tied to a much larger community system of controls and accountability are often used by assailants to get back into their homes, to win court and custody battles, to avoid criminal and civil court sanctions and proceedings, and to convince their partners that they are changing, even when there is no true altering of the power dynamics in the relationship.

A community needs to use its institutional powers to confront batterers and make a commitment to place increasingly harsh penalties and sanctions on men who continue to abuse their partners. To conduct men's groups without having first insisted on services for battered women and on police and court reforms is not only shortsighted, but in the long run, also dangerous to some battered women.

An essential factor in the success of the Duluth intervention model has been the support of the judicial system. Ninety-two percent of the abusers convicted in Duluth of assaulting their partners are court mandated to the DAIP. Twelve percent have served some jail time as a consequence of their abuse. Ninety-seven percent of all civil protection orders granted in cases in which minor children are involved also carry a mandate to attend batterers' groups conducted by the DAIP.

Today the primary functions of the DAIP are to monitor the compliance of agencies in the community with agreed-on policies and to monitor individual batterers' compliance with court orders. Monitoring the response of police, prosecutors, and other agencies involved occurs through a continual review of records and periodic interviews with victims. The DAIP monitors individuals through reviewing the records of counseling agencies and of groups conducted by the DAIP and through frequent contacts and interviews with the individual's partner.

To allow for communication between the counseling agencies and the DAIP, all batterers court ordered to a rehabilitation program are ordered directly to the DAIP. The assailant signs both an interagency release of information (the DAIP is defined as an interagency team) to allow participating agencies to share information and a rehabilitation contract that clearly describes each man's obligations under the court order (Appendix 3). After completing an intake and orientation session, he is assigned to one of the ongoing 24-week groups conducted by community therapists or educators.

The monitoring and coordinating role of the DAIP is intended to prevent community collusion with abusers. It ensures that individual police officers, probation officers, therapists, prosecutors, judges, advocates, and jailers are not screening cases out of the system based on misinformation provided by the abuser; lack of information; or race, gender, or class bias. Such screening is one of the most common ways communities collude with abusers.

Every aspect of community intervention—developing an intake process, using jail, excluding batterers from their homes, implementing a group rehabilitation process—communicates a message to those battering and those being battered. The DAIP is an independent organization strongly influenced by formerly battered women, which, through bimonthly interagency meetings, provides a vehicle for open discussion about the daily operation of the intervention process and about ways of improving our collective response. When the project functions properly, each case is open to scrutiny. Each case can be held up for examination and accountability. The system then is not conducive to collusion.

THE DAIP MEN'S PROGRAM DESIGN

Figure 2.1 illustrates the intervention process set in motion by a court referral to the program.

Court Referral

Criminal court probation agreements require that each assailant contact the DAIP within 5 working days of his sentencing hearing to set up an appointment for an intake. These agreements state the expectation that the assailant will complete the 26-week program under the rules of the DAIP.

Civil protection order hearings are held once a week. A DAIP staff person attends these hearings and, after the judge has issued an order, meets with the man to explain the program and assign an intake date. Like criminal court probation agreements, the civil court order specifically requires respondents to cooperate completely with the DAIP and to complete the program. It is important that both probation agreements and civil protection orders spell out the obligations of assailants. Clear and specific language leaves fewer loopholes for batterers who are brought back to court for failure to comply with court orders.

DAIP Flow Chart

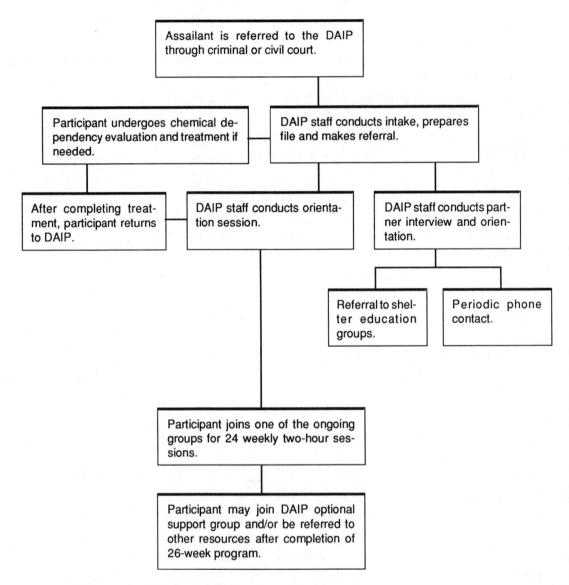

Figure 2.1 Flow chart of intervention process.

Intake

In most cases intake sessions are conducted with groups of 6 to 10 men the week following their court appearance. If more than 10 men are court ordered to the DAIP in a week, a second session is scheduled. We moved from hour-long individual intakes to 3-hour-long group intakes in 1990, primarily to save time. It soon became clear to us, however, that there were many advantages to the group intake process.

Ty

I resisted the idea of group intakes for a long time. It just seemed too impersonal, like herding cattle, prodding the men from this group to the next group without ever really talking to them. I wanted at least one private session with each guy so that he could know that someone took the time to listen to his whole story. Finally I agreed to try one or two group intakes and I was absolutely amazed at the difference. I think the men looked around and saw six or seven other guys all court ordered to the program, and some let down their defenses. With individual intakes the men are much more defensive. Almost every word they utter is either victim blaming or justification for their violence. So I have to start confronting all of that stuff right from the beginning and it gets very intense. The group intakes are totally different.

It's best when two of us conduct the intake. One does the interviewing and the other records the information on the intake form. We usually switch off and interview every other man in the group.

In the intake process the interviewer probes for the following information from each man:

- The pattern and severity of his violence toward his current partner, past partners, his children, other acquaintances, and strangers. This information is used to assess the danger level to the woman he has abused and to those who are intervening to stop him.
- His level of openness and honesty about his use of violence. We can compare his comments to the police report or the protection order papers in his file. These reports give fairly detailed accounts by victims and police officers of at least one violent incident.
- His history of drugs, alcohol, and mental health problems. This information is used to determine if any specialized assessments should be made a part of his contract.
- The likelihood that he will be disruptive in groups. This is used to determine if he should be assigned to a group for men who are either in complete denial that they are violent or unwilling to make a commitment to change.

- The likelihood that he will engage in self-destructive behaviors or become suicidal or homicidal. The interviewer probes for this information to encourage men to use counselors from mental health agencies associated with the DAIP if they need individual counseling in addition to their educational groups.
- Any special needs he may have to complete groups successfully. About 7% of the men we work with cannot read or write, and another 15% have very poor writing skills. Ten percent of court-mandated men work in the Great Lakes shipping industry, in the trucking industry, or in jobs requiring them to be gone for weeks at a time. Arrangements for such absences are made and special conditions put in men's contracts.
- His awareness of the services available to him in the community. Many men are unaware of the special services of the Vet Center, the Visitation Center (which offers supervised visitiation and a neutral site for parents who are separated or divorced to drop off and pick up their children), groups for parents of children who have witnessed battering, and other services of use to people with a history of violence in relationships.
- His use of violence toward his children and, often, the visitation and custody arrangements regarding his children. This information is obtained to assess the need for protective measures for the children and to be aware of what measures have already been taken in that regard.
- His understanding of his contract and the interagency release of information he will sign with his contract. Because of the possibility of his being sent back to court for failure to complete the program or follow the rules, it is important that we are assured that he fully understands his obligations at the time he enters the program.

The facilitators discuss the philosophy of the program by describing the Power and Control and Equality Wheels and show the video *Profile of an Assailant*.[2] In this film a former batterer describes his violence, his efforts to blame his partner and his eventual decision to change.

Between 11 and 15 men's groups meet on a weekly basis in Duluth. A man is assigned to one of the open-ended groups in progress based on the space available and the schedule that is most convenient for the participant. Each man is required to attend 24 sessions. He is allowed two absences during the first 12 weeks and another two during the second 12 weeks. All absences must be made up.

Following the intake, the DAIP staff prepares a file containing a summary of the police report, intake information, notations from the probation officer, the history of abuse the victim wants the counselor to know about, and a summary of the assailant's self-reported past violence. For various reasons, about 7% of the men who are court mandated to the DAIP have individual intakes in addition to or instead of group intakes. The same information is obtained in the individual intake although the intake often focuses on the particular problem which made the individual intake necessary (e.g., drug and alcohol problems, history of mental illness, scheduling problems).

SCREENING PARTICIPANTS

It has been the practice of the DAIP to accept almost anyone mandated by the courts. The project also accepts most voluntary participants. Individuals are rarely screened out.

For various reasons, however, some participants are inappropriate for group. This decision is made by the men's program coordinator either at intake or when problems surface during participation in group.

- *Alcohol or drug abuse:* Occasionally a participant may have a chemical abuse problem that does not become apparent until after he has entered the program. If the problem surfaces in group, the facilitator reports the participant to the men's program coordinator, who then usually requests an evaluation. If the participant refuses, he can be ordered back to the court. (Voluntary participants may be terminated from the program.) Men with chronic or severe alcohol or drug problems may not be appropriate for group. The reality is, however, that more than half of the group members will be using excessive amounts of alcohol or drugs, which requires some flexibility on program admittance.
- *Psychological problems:* Individual therapy sometimes is required in addition to batterers' groups but is rarely ordered in lieu of the DAIP program. Most group members are participating not because of a personal or family dysfunction but rather because violence is a socialized option for men. To attach a clinical diagnosis to the batterer's use of violence provides a rationalization for behavior that may not be accurate. There are individuals, however, who have psychological problems that make their involvement in groups difficult and counterproductive to the rest of the group. Psychiatric or neurological evaluations are ordered by the court if the incidents seem to warrant investigation by appropriate mental health personnel. If mental illness is diagnosed and an abuser's illness prevents him from participating in group, other treatment may be required. However, this occurs infrequently.
- *Disruptive behavior:* If a participant is continually disruptive in the group, but he has not committed a new offense, missed groups, or failed to complete written assignments, the facilitator can, for the sake of the group process, refer him back to the program coordinator to be transferred into a group entirely made up of men unwilling to work in groups. If his disruption goes beyond a negative or hostile

attitude, he can be referred back to court for noncompliance with the court order. These two options are important for the mental health of facilitators and for creating a positive climate for men who want to make changes. In the group for disruptive men, the structure is more lecture oriented than is this curriculum.

Confidentiality and Participants' Files

Participants entering a batterers' program are required to sign a release of information. Through it, contact with a participant's partner is permitted and his file is available to the DAIP team of group facilitators, therapists, chemical dependency counselors, and representatives of the court or corrections who have a relationship with the participant because of probation or a civil protection order. Participants refusing to sign the release are not allowed to participate and are referred back to the court.

The participant is informed through the contract he signs that the program will contact his partner to obtain a history of abuse, that she will also be given the name of the counselor or facilitator he is working with, and that she will be notified of any pending court hearings regarding his involvement in the program. Again, if he refuses to sign, he is not allowed into the program. These conditions are requirements for voluntary participants as well as for court-mandated individuals.

Participants' files are kept separate from the victims' reports because participants have the right to examine their own files. Under no circumstances should a batterer have access to reports of his partner's calls or comments. Because under some circumstances a participant is able to subpoena his partner's file, which would give him access to her calls and comments to facilitators, program staff must be cautious about what information is recorded in partners' files.

Voluntary Participants

Individuals volunteer to participate in groups for a variety of reasons. Some men volunteer immediately following an assault because they are afraid of the potential legal implications of their violence. Some men believe that entering the program voluntarily will lessen the penalty if their case enters the court system. Some are fearful that their partners will leave them, so they seek help. Others are truly remorseful and are willing to change at any cost. The reality at the DAIP is that only 10% of all men who come in to volunteer for the groups complete the 26-week program.

One reason few volunteers complete the program may be the curriculum itself, because it challenges the participant's long-held beliefs. Another reason may be that voluntary participants are treated the same as those who are court mandated, and must follow the same rules on participation, assignments, and attendance. Treating volunteers differently because they have volunteered minimizes their violence and sets them apart from the men who were brought into the group through the court system.

Voluntary participants entering the program sign a contract outlining the same obligations to the program as court-ordered men. Volunteers are informed that if they leave the program, their partners will be notified. About half of the time when we notify a woman that her abuser has stopped his voluntary participation, she tells us that he has threatened or committed another act of violence or that she has informed him she is leaving the relationship. The woman often decides at this point to get a civil protection order and the voluntary participant who has dropped out is now court mandated to the program and must start the program over.

Men's Orientation Session

The orientation session is the second group participants attend. Like the intake, it is conducted by the men's program coordinator. The following agenda describes the session:

- Each man introduces himself and gives a brief explanation of how he got into the program.
- Group rules are explained.
- The eight themes of the curriculum are described.
    - Theme One: Nonviolence
    - Theme Two: Nonthreatening Behavior
    - Theme Three: Respect
    - Theme Four: Support and Trust
    - Theme Five: Accountability and Honesty
    - Theme Six: Sexual Respect
    - Theme Seven: Partnership
    - Theme Eight: Negotiation and Fairness
- The control log and the action plan are introduced with a brief explanation of how they are used in group.
- The program coordinator talks briefly about the need for men to use the groups to focus on themselves rather than on their partners or their problems with the courts or visitation.

The week after a participant finishes his orientation session, he attends his first group. He may be joining the group during the second or third week of a theme. This is preferable to his waiting several weeks to start the program at the beginning of a theme.

PARTNER CONTACTS

Most programs that offer groups for men who batter have some contact with each participant's partner. Our purpose in contacting women is to obtain a history of her partner's abuse, invite her to an orientation session, and provide her information on resources available in the community. DAIP staff do not elicit information from partners until safety planning has been explored and the propriety of using the information is determined.

Women's Orientation

DAIP staff attempts to contact by phone the partner of each participant in the program to get her assessment of abuse in the relationship. The women's program coordinator invites her to attend two women's orientation sessions and an ongoing support group. If the woman can't be reached by phone, a letter is sent.

In part, these sessions are designed to give the partner an overview of the men's program because a participant may lie or intentionally distort information from groups and his facilitators and present it to his partner as proof that she is to blame for the "relationship problems." He can prove it because he now has some sophisticated language he learned in group.

At the orientation sessions, the women's program coordinator discusses the following:

- The men's program, including an explanation or the Power and Control Wheel, the goals of the program, and the structure of the curriculum.
- The Abusive Behavior Inventory (Appendix 4), a tool for women to assess any changes their partners may be making. It is a questionnaire designed to help women assess over time whether their partners are significantly reducing all forms of abusive behavior or merely complying with their probation or court agreements not to use illegal acts of violence and increasing the use of legal tactics of control. (This questionnaire is also used as the basis for our ongoing evaluation of the program.)
- Safety issues as well as protective options available to women, such as orders for protection; the Visitation Center; revocation of probation or review of protection orders; hearings; and shelter services, including legal advocacy.

Women are encouraged to participate in ongoing neighborhood-based educational programs, the Indian Women's Talking Circle, or the Women's Action Group, which works on furthering the institutional changes occurring in Duluth related to issues of poverty and violence against women and children.

CONCLUSION

This chapter has provided an overview of the DAIP and has discussed the essential role of the community agencies involved. We would not offer batterers' groups without the involvement of these agencies in the community's response to battering. The fundamental principle that guides this project continues to be safety for battered women.

NOTES

1. A complete description of this interagency model, including policies of all participating agencies, is contained in the manual *Criminal Justice Response to Domestic Assault: A Guide for Policy Development*, available through DAIP's National Training Project. For information on ordering it or other DAIP materials referred to in this book, please contact the DAIP's National Training Project, 206 West 4th Street, Duluth, MN 55806.

2. *Profile of an Assailant* is available from the DAIP's National Training Project (see above note).

Chapter 3

The Curriculum

CURRICULUM DESIGN

In 1984 the DAIP moved from anger management and Batterers Anonymous groups to an educational and counseling approach that focused on the use of violence by a batterer to establish power and control over his partner. We designed and developed a curriculum to ensure more consistency in how groups were structured and conducted.

Based on our experience, we wanted the curriculum to accomplish the following:

- Ensure that women's reality and women's experiences were always a part of the group content.
- Account for cultural and social diversity in the group and explain the impact of socialization on the use of violence.
- Keep the facilitator from getting caught up in all of the personal problems the men are facing.
- Keep the men focused for 2 hours in each group on themselves and their use of violence against women, rather than on their partners or relationships.
- Help the men practice ways to change their behavior.

To do all of this we created several tools for facilitators to use in groups. Most of those tools are contained in this book, including control logs, action plans, outlines of the video vignettes/role plays, and descriptions of group exercises. While designing the curriculum we worked with a local television station to tape 13 short vignettes and a series of discussions among battered women. We also taped a men's group to demonstrate the use of the control log, described later in this chapter.

These videos are available to readers who attend trainings sponsored by the DAIP's National Training Project.[1] For those who do not have access to the videos we have written role plays that take their place.

The video vignettes or role plays are 3- to 5-minute dramatizations of incidents related in women's groups as examples of the use of tactics on the Power and Control Wheel.

Objectives of Curriculum

The curriculum is designed to help men stop battering by achieving five objectives.

- To assist the participant to understand that his acts of violence are a means of controlling his partner's actions, thoughts, and feelings by examining the intent of his acts of abuse and the belief system from which he operates.
- To increase the participant's understanding of the causes of his violence by examining the cultural and social contexts in which he uses violence against his partner.
- To increase the participant's willingness to change his actions by examining the negative effects of his behavior on his relationship, his partner, his children, his friends, and himself.
- To encourage the participant to become accountable to those he has hurt through his use of violence by helping him to acknowledge his abuse, accept responsibility for its impact on his partner and others, and take specific steps to change.
- To provide the participant with practical information on how to change abusive behavior by exploring noncontrolling and nonviolent ways of relating to women.

Themes of Curriculum

The curriculum is based on eight themes, each of which is explored over a 3-week period. Each theme represents an aspect of nonviolent and respectful relationships.

The eight themes are depicted on the Equality Wheel (see Figure 3.1). The behaviors and aspects of an egalitarian relationship shown on the wheel become the model offered to men for egalitarian and interdependent relationships with women.

The Power and Control Wheel (see Figure 3.2) depicts the primary tactics and behaviors individual abusers use to establish and maintain control in their relationships.

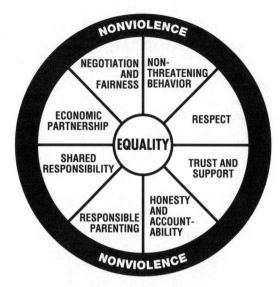

Figure 3.1   Equality Wheel.

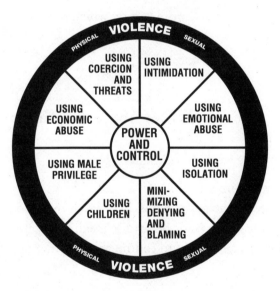

Figure 3.2   Power and Control Wheel.

THREE-WEEK OUTLINE

The following is an overview of the structure of the 3 weeks of each theme and a description of the teaching tools used.

Week 1:
Defining the Theme and Analyzing Specific Abusive Behavior

There are five activities for week 1 of a theme.

- The group begins with check-in, in which men briefly discuss progress toward the goals on their action plans. (Some programs use this curriculum to teach large classes of 30 to 35 men and do not use a check-in process.)
- The group defines the theme on the Equality Wheel to be explained. For example, what does it mean to trust and support a partner?
- The group analyzes a 3- to 5-minute video or role play of a story that depicts a man using a tactic on the Power and Control Wheel that is in contrast to the behavior on the Equality Wheel (e.g., trust). The group uses the seven-part control log to analyze the scene.
- The facilitator gives a brief lecture about the many forms and impact of the tactic being discussed.
- The facilitator distributes control logs on which participants record and analyze an abusive incident.

Week 2:
Examining Specific Acts of Abuse as a Tactic of Control

There are two activities in week 2 of a theme.

- The group begins with check-in.
- The group analyzes the participants' logs. Each man's log identifies a personal example of his use of the tactic being discussed. For example, the men will log a time when they used isolation to control their partner or a former partner.

Week 3:
Exploring and Practicing Noncontrolling and Nonviolent Behavior

There are three activities for Week 3 of a theme.

- The group begins with check-in.
- Several group members role play noncontrolling alternatives to abusive incidents from their own control logs.

- The group uses exercises to learn skills based on issues that have surfaced during the previous 2 weeks. The exercises deal with taking time-outs, acknowledging women's fear, accepting women's anger, using positive self-talk, being assertive rather than aggressive, recognizing nonverbal cues, communicating feelings and thoughts, negotiating, and letting go.

TEACHING TOOLS

Each week of the curriculum uses teaching tools designed to focus the group on the very difficult and complex issue of men's violence toward women. The *check-in* is used at the beginning of each session, in which men identify specific steps they are taking toward change. They record these steps on their *action plans*. Then during the first week, the group analyzes a short *video or role play* using a *control log*. The second week requires men to explore their own use of abusive behaviors, again using the control log, and the third week they practice alternative nonviolent behaviors in *role plays* and *group exercises*.

Check-Ins

Most counseling and education groups have something similar to a check-in. This is the introduction to a group session.

Unfortunately, check-ins often become time-consuming discussions about issues unrelated to the reasons for participants being in the group. Group members will discuss their having become angry at work, their cars breaking down, their fishing trips, and their general frames of mind. A check-in that runs this course becomes an avoidance strategy indirectly condoned by facilitators.

When using this curriculum, facilitators limit the check-in to reporting on the men's action plans, disclosing use of violence or abuse during the previous week, and introducing new members.

Action Plan

The action plan (see Table 3.1 and Appendix 5) is a written record of the goals and steps to which participants commit themselves while in the program. The goals and the steps must be concrete and realistic and should be focused on changing specific controlling or abusive behaviors whether or not the participant is still living with the woman he abused.

The facilitators use a flipchart to write each man's first name, goals, and steps to achieve those goals. During the 24-week program, each man will always have at least one goal on the action plan.

During week 2 (control logs) or week 3 (noncontrolling behaviors) a participant may realize he wants to add something to his action plan, and the facilitator records it on the flipchart. New goals are added on a weekly basis.

Identification of Action Plan Goals and Steps

During the course of analyzing the vignettes or role plays and logging the men's examples of using controlling or abusive behavior, participants make personal disclosures about aspects of their past, their attitudes about women, their family and relationships, and present issues and problems. When a participant raises an issue he needs to work on,

Table 3.1

Weekly Group Action Plan

Changes I am making	Steps to take
Harold	
Be respectful of my partner	Think about all my interactions with her at the end of the day. Stop using sarcasm. Don't blame her for my negativism. Try fair-fighting concepts. Stop using intimidation. Don't talk when she's already saying something.
Warren	
Stop invading her privacy	Don't check up on her by asking the kids what she's up to. Don't drive by her house or her place of work. Leave it up to her as to when she wants phone contact.
Steve	
Stop picking fights so I can leave the house	Talk to her about wanting to spend time with my friends. Take responsibility for finding childcare on nights I want to go out. Quit making a big deal of it when she goes out.

the facilitators propose making this a goal for him to work toward and, with his consent, place it on the weekly action plan.

The following is an example of how goals are identified and how the action plan is used.

FACILITATOR: Craig, when we were discussing how you used male privilege to avoid helping Carol with the kids, you said that the effect on the relationship was that Carol would get angry and resentful.

CRAIG: Yeah, things would get pretty cold. And I'm not really sure why I got into this rut with her. I'd come home from work tired and lay down on the couch and watch TV, and she'd get pissed.

FACILITATOR: From your log it looks like you understand why she would be angry with you.

CRAIG: I knew at the time that what I was doing was pissing her off but whenever she'd bring it up I'd get defensive, you know, and argue that I had a right to relax after working all day. And she'd say, "What about my work all day?" Then I'd say the two can't be compared and we'd be off to the races.

FACILITATOR: On the effects section you said that one effect on you was that you missed time with your children. Do you still feel that loss?

CRAIG: Yeah.

FACILITATOR: Would you be willing to commit to a goal on your action plan where you take a bigger role in child care and free Carol up a little?

CRAIG: I'd be willing.

FACILITATOR: Any suggestions from the group for Craig in coming up with steps to make this goal happen?

JEFF: You could spend time with the kids as soon as you get home and watch TV later.

TONY: You could work out some kind of plan with Carol so it's more of a compromise.

FACILITATOR: Let's list a couple of these steps and we'll see how they worked during check-in next week.

If the participant is not currently in a relationship, the goals on his action plan could include not harassing his ex-partner, not saying negative things about his ex-partner to his children, letting go of obsessive thoughts about her, getting on with his life, and examining negative attitudes toward women.

Control Log

The control log (see Figure 3.3 and Appendix 6) is a primary teaching tool of this curriculum. It is designed to facilitate a group analysis of six key elements of an abusive act and then to define alternatives to those acts. The six elements include naming behaviors that constitute abusive action, identifying the intent of the abuser in using that action and the underlying belief system that justified it, identifying feelings that motivated him to act, examining the impact of his actions on the woman he abused and on others in his life,

CONTROL LOG

Men's Education Groups

Name **_John_**

Date **_July 19th_**

1. ACTIONS: Briefly describe the situation and the actions you used to control your partner (statements, gestures, tone of voice, physical contact, facial expressions).

   Grabbed her by her hair — called her names, — slammed door.

2. INTENTS AND BELIEFS: What did you want to happen in this situation?

   For her to stop swearing at me and to quit yelling.

   What beliefs do you have that support your actions and intents?

   It takes two to tango.

3. FEELINGS: What feelings were you having?

   Mad, frustrated

4. MINIMIZATION, DENIAL AND BLAME: In what ways did you minimize or deny your actions or blame her?

   She spit at me, that's why I had to grab her.

5. EFFECTS: What was the impact of your action?

   On you **_spent the night in the car_**

   On her **_she's scared_**

   On others **_kids woke up crying_**

6. PAST VIOLENCE: How did your past use of violence affect this situation?

   Made her afraid, she went to the courts.

7. NON-CONTROLLING BEHAVIORS: What could you have done differently?

   I should have left as soon as she started yelling at me.

Figure 3.3

and acknowledging the relationship of his past use of violence to his action and his partner's reaction to him. Finally, the log assists in exploring nonviolent, noncontrolling ways of dealing with conflict in a relationship.

The log is used throughout the curriculum. It is the framework for discussion of each of the eight themes and is intended to maintain a continual focus on the participants' behavior, excluding from discussion rationalizations, victim blaming, and opportunities for collusion. It thus alleviates some of the pressure on the facilitators to confront abusive behavior, as it makes the entire session a confrontation.

The log is also used to analyze the 13 videos or role-played stories described earlier. Using the log allows men to look objectively at how and why abusive tactics are used in relationships. During the analysis of the scenes the groups frequently discuss the forces that influence men's lives, the values men are socialized to have, and the costs of this socialization to them and to women who are victims of male violence.

In the second week of each theme the logs are used to examine the participants' own personal experiences. The participants' resistance to acknowledging their own behaviors makes this session far more difficult to facilitate. One facilitator described the difference between how the men log the videotaped scene and how they log their personal examples as follows:

Wendy

They show the man in the film no mercy. His every move, glance and word is analyzed and exposed as controlling or abusive. The next week, as the men put their own behaviors on the board, all of a sudden everyone in the group seems to lose his clarity about what those behaviors were intended to accomplish.

The group analysis of the video or role play provides an important foundation for the next week's session when the men look at their own behaviors. Again, one of the facilitators offers a comment on this point.

Scott

When the group is asked to list reasons why the man in the video did something, they are really very good at seeing how often he is abusing her to get power or to get her to do or think something that benefits him. But when we start analyzing their own behaviors, everything gets confused and lots of times I get this sinking feeling that I don't know where to go with the conversation. It starts getting into how their partners nag or manipulate and how spontaneous their responses are. It really helps me and the group when I can just say, "Wait a minute, how about last week's discussion on smashing things? Last week we all said it was for power, now suddenly this week it's an uncontrollable response. Why?" That helps. The first week really allows for a somewhat detached discussion on what all these actions are really about. It helps later, when the discussion becomes personal.

The third week focuses solely on section 7 of the log. Using a combination of role plays acted out by the men, lectures, and exercises, the men explore and practice noncontrolling behavior.

Each section of the log facilitates an examination of an important element of battering. To look thoroughly at any of these elements, the group needs to focus its discussion in a given session on one or two sections in the control log while briefly covering the remaining sections. If the group spends only 5 to 10 minutes on each section, the process will degenerate into a superficial exercise in list making. The facilitator learns to sense when to pursue an issue and on which of the sections to focus the group's attention. Over a 24-week period, each section of the control log will have been the intense focus of the group's discussion during several sessions.

The log to be examined subsequently was turned in by one of the participants in a DAIP group during week 2 of a theme. It is presented here in sections, each followed by an explanation of the group's objectives in examining that section and the process used to meet them. The first of these sections is presented in Figure 3.4.

Actions

1. ACTIONS: Briefly describe the situation and the actions you used to control your partner (statements, gestures, tone of voice, physical contact, facial expressions).

Grabbed her by her hair — called her names, — slammed door.

Figure 3.4 Example of action section of control log.

Objectives

The group's objectives in examining the action section of the log follow:

1. To examine the pattern that individuals use in controlling their partners.
2. To reduce minimizing their behaviors by putting them in a larger context.
3. To challenge the claim "I just blew" by helping the men see how they use a complex system of behaviors.
4. To illustrate that there are numerous controlling and abusive actions within one incident.

Process

A key word here is "briefly." Group members will often fill this section in with an excuse for being controlling: "My wife was nagging me all day long so I finally yelled at her," or

"My wife was going out to see a guy she'd been running around with so I pulled the distributor cap out of her car."

In recording the report on the board, the facilitator omits the editorial comment and focuses on the behavior—"Pulled out distributor cap."

In a small group the facilitator may choose to log one man's example. In a large group the facilitator quickly goes around the room and records one example of an abusive action from each participant, focusing on one or two men's examples to draw out more details.

In the action section, the participant logs only controlling behavior. He will have a tendency to give a thumbnail sketch of what occurred. For example, he may say, "My wife called me a name so I got angry." Getting angry is not necessarily an action used to gain control. If he threw something or punched a wall or swore at her, calling her names and intimidating her, that is the controlling action. Before moving on to the next section, detail as much of the participant's actions as practical. For example;

FACILITATOR: You said that you began yelling at her. What exactly did you say? What names did you call her?
Did you move toward her?
Did you throw things in her direction or break things?

Sometimes a man's example does not illustrate controlling behavior. If he uses an example of his wife being abusive, the facilitator needs to confront him on his refusal to look at his own behavior. When this happens, the facilitator should ask him to fill out a log on an incident in which he was controlling before he leaves the group that week.

Before moving on to the next section, summarize by identifying which combinations of controlling tactics on the Power and Control Wheel the participant used. This demonstrates the interconnectedness of these tactics, which form a pattern of behaviors, rather than exist as isolated incidents.

Intents and Beliefs

Figure 3.5 presents the intents and beliefs section of the log.

2. INTENTS AND BELIEFS: What did you want to happen in this situation?
For her to stop swearing at me and to quit yelling.

What beliefs do you have that support your actions and intents?
It takes two to tango.

Figure 3.5 Example of intents and beliefs section of control log.

Objectives

The group's objectives in examining the intents and beliefs section of the log follow:

1. To acknowledge the function of battering.
2. To acknowledge that these behaviors are not out of control but are intentional acts to establish control.
3. To examine the many societal and personal experiences that have shaped men's values and beliefs about men and women and intimate relationships.
4. To name and understand the source of many beliefs that support and justify abusive behavior.

Process

The facilitator poses questions regarding the intents of actions on two levels. The first is to explore the intents of specific behaviors (e.g., intimidating stares, throwing or smashing objects, name calling, driving recklessly) and the second is to ask what he wanted to achieve by *all* of his actions in a given situation.

Exploration of intents of specific tactics

Frequently the participants will report their intentions as honorable or at least understandable (e.g., "I was trying to keep her from getting hurt by her mother so . . ."). The facilitator may wish to probe further by asking a few questions, but generally a man's statement of intent is related to what he wanted to have happen as a result of his actions: "I was trying to keep her from going to her mother's." The group first examines the intent of the words, body language and gestures that were used. The following is an example from a group of 18 men.

FACILITATOR: Here's the list of all the ways or words that people have said they use to put their partners down or attack them emotionally: slut, bitch, fat, bad mother, tramp. . . . Let's look at some of this in context. By that I mean, I don't suppose, Joe, when you called her a slut you were sitting back relaxed in a nonthreatening posture using a soft tender voice?

JOE: No, I don't suppose that either.

FACILITATOR: Describe for the group what your tone was.

JOE: Well, I guess my tone was gruff.

FACILITATOR: You guess? Or was it?

JOE: Yeah, it was. I didn't think I made any moves toward her. I pretty much just called her a slut.

FACILITATOR: Okay, Joe, let's you and I act this out to get a better idea of it.

JOE: How about we don't?

FACILITATOR: Look at it this way, if you act it out for 2 minutes now, I won't ask you to do it next week when you'd have to role play the whole scene.

JOE: OK. (He stands up.) I was standing. She was sitting.

FACILITATOR: Where am I? (The scene is acted out.)

FACILITATOR: How about observations? Kyle, what actions did you see that went hand in hand with the words?

KYLE: He was pretty intimidating.

FACILITATOR: Tell Joe directly. (Facilitators constantly need to prompt the men to talk directly to each other rather than addressing their remarks to the facilitator when discussing role plays.)

KYLE: You were pretty intimidating with your body and the way you grabbed your jacket.

FACILITATOR: Jack, what about you? Did you see anything else that went with Joe's words?

JACK: His tone. He said it was gruff—it might have been a bit more than gruff to her.

FACILITATOR: (Points to Joe.)

JACK: (Directing his remark to Joe.) You're a big guy. I'm sure that put a scare into her.

This process puts all the participants' actions on the board, but focuses on one or two men to bring out the patterns and details.

The group goes on to examine intents.

FACILITATOR: OK. Let's look at the intent for using these names. It seems almost half of you are using names such as slut, tramp, whore. Let's look at that first. How do these names affect a woman?

The group discusses how making women into sex objects and then defining sex objects as bad degrades women and lowers their self-esteem. From there the group goes on to discuss why men would want women to have low self-esteem. Again, the facilitator brings the discussion back to an intent identified by a group member.

FACILITATOR: Sam, we're talking about women's self-esteem, and you said your intent was to "get her to see how she was acting." Was part of that to get her to dislike how she was acting?

SAM: Sure. It wasn't a good way to act.

FACILITATOR: So, she's acting a way you don't like and you want her to share your opinion of her behavior?

SAM: Yes. To see how dumb it was.

FACILITATOR: So, if she thought what you wanted her to think, what would happen?

SAM: She'd stop doing it.

FACILITATOR: Why? Because she'd be embarrassed?

SAM: Sure.

FACILITATOR: Do you see the connection between making her feel bad about herself and getting her to act the way you want?

SAM: Yes.

FACILITATOR: How about you, Frank? Do you see a connection?

FRANK: Sure. That's what I'm doing—calling her dumb or stupid so she'll quit doing something. You know, it kind of shakes up her confidence. Makes her more reserved.

In this way, the group members collectively analyze their experiences on the log.

Exploration of the overall intent of an abusive action

The second level of examining the intent of abusive acts is to identify the purpose of the entire exchange (e.g., to keep her from getting a job, to get her to be quiet).

In examining this second level of intents the facilitator is looking for a common ground for group members to begin a discussion. For example, if participants watch the vignette or role play on the story *I'm Just Asking a Couple of Simple Questions* (Chapter 5, Theme Four), and several men agree that Steve's intent in picking a fight and stomping out was to give himself an excuse to go out, get drunk, and stay out all night, then the group needs to go one step further. Why pick a fight, scare her, and get all worked up just so he can go out and get drunk? Because so many men have done this, the question prompts a discussion about feeling trapped in a relationship but not wanting one's partner to be able to go out all night. So the man picks a fight. This discussion can take many directions. The facilitator is not required to determine the conclusion but to keep in front of the group questions about fairness, double standards, abusive tactics, exploitation, and objectification of their partners. How does the discussion ultimately relate to why a man wants a woman in his life? What does he see as her role, and is that a fair expectation?

Exploration of beliefs

This section usually generates the most discussion and reflection. The discussion of beliefs emerges from the discussion on intents. In the following discussion, a facilitator refers to the vignette/role play *You Don't Care About What I Need* (Chapter 5, Theme Two).

FACILITATOR: If we're saying that Steve slammed down the checkbook, ripped the phone out of the wall, yelled at Cathy, and stormed out of the house to punish her for not taking care of him, then what is one belief Steve holds that supports all of this?

JACK: It's her job.

RANDY: She's supposed to know what he needs and plan for him if she loves him.

TOM: Love means you never have to take care of yourself. (Laughter from the group.)

These belief statements bring the group to the discussion about societal values and the socialization of men and women. How did Steve come to believe this? Is it natural or cultural? This presents the opportunity for the facilitator to teach theory by using a drawing of a pyramid to relate Jack's comments to the structure of hierarchy.

The concept that the natural order of things is hierarchical is important to explore with the men because it is at the heart of their belief in their natural right to be in charge and, therefore, to set and enforce rules and roles. A drawing of a pyramid is frequently used in exploring variations of this theme.

The following is an exercise that can be used to illustrate hierarchy. After drawing a pyramid on the board, ask the group members to think of an organization that has had an impact on them, for example, their place of work, the military, a social club, the welfare system, a school or their family of origin. Next ask the following questions:

- Who is at the top of the pyramid?
- How did he or she get there?
- Are they there because they are the most talented or because they work the hardest?
- Who is immediately under him or her?
- Who is at the bottom?
- Who is in the middle?
- Where in that system is each man in the group?

Looking at the hierarchical system in terms of their workplace, the service, school, or church gives the men a way of examining systems removed from their family situations. Aspects for discussion regarding these systems include the following:

- How do people at the bottom of the hierarchy influence those at the top to get what they want and need? (This question may also generate discussion on the belief of many batterers that women are manipulative, discussed in Chapter 2.)
- How must people act to move up in this hierarchy?
- How have they benefited from or been hurt by the hierarchy that they are in?
- What would happen if the workplace had a more democratic system for decision making?
- Would it improve the product?
- Would it create more motivation among the workers?
- How were the families the men grew up in structured?
- Again the facilitator draws a pyramid and asks the participants where they were in the pyramid. Where were each man's father, mother, older brother, and younger sisters on the pyramid? What was the impact of these hierarchical relationships on individuals in the family?

Throughout the 24 weeks discussions will emerge that can best be understood by returning to the image of the pyramid and asking questions about the relationship of this discussion to the hierarchical or authoritarian context in which the situation is occurring.

The discussion of beliefs is at the heart of helping men think critically about how they want to lead their lives and what they want in an intimate relationship with a woman. It moves them from a spontaneous reaction ("That's the way it's supposed to be") to a thoughtful look at how things could be. If the nature of the relationship is to change, the system and the beliefs that support it must change.

When the participants in the group make statements such as "Men are paychecks to women," the facilitator can focus discussion on the beliefs that support those statements. In using the curriculum, beliefs are explored for two purposes.

- To give participants insight about a belief that supports the use of violence or abusive behaviors.
- To give participants suggestions on steps they can take to change their patterns of abusive behaviors.

These beliefs may surface at any point in the group discussion, but the facilitator specifically draws them out during the discussion on intents by asking the second question in this section, "What beliefs do you have that support your actions and intents?"

Exploring a belief entails four steps.

1. Formulating a *belief or problem statement* based on group discussion.
2. Exploring different *aspects for discussion* of that belief statement, particularly the implications of that belief to sustaining authoritarian hierarchical relationships.
3. Exploring its *relationship to the use of violence* or other abusive behaviors.
4. Naming *ways to eliminate related violence* and abusive behaviors.

Step 1. Belief or problem statement. During the first step, the facilitator focuses on statements made by a group member and then poses a problem or a belief statement it suggests. For example:

> BILL: That's the way it was in my family. That's the way it was in my dad's family. The man brought home the paycheck, and the woman took care of the house.
>
> FACILITATOR: Bill, let's go into that a little deeper. Families have traditionally been set up in a way that divides labor—the man works outside the home for money, and the woman works in the home but doesn't get paid. What are the effects of that kind of setup, whether it is the man working outside the home or the woman working outside the home, on the balance of power between the man and woman in their personal relationship?

In this case the facilitator has posed the problem of the power imbalance that results when one person brings home a paycheck and the other provides free labor at home. The purpose of exploring this problem is to look at how this situation leads to power imbalance and the potential for violence and then to name some specific steps that can prevent it.

Step 2. Aspects for discussion. Once the facilitator has posed the problem or belief, the group discusses various aspects of that statement. Examples of questions might be: "How do we come to believe this?" "Who benefits by these beliefs?" and "If this is true, what else is true?"

In the case of Bill talking about men bringing home the paycheck, the group talked about what it would be like if their partners worked outside the home, and they did not. This actually was the situation for several of the men. They listed the pros and cons of being the one to stay home.

FACILITATOR: If we were to look at these two lists, the things we think are positive and the things we think are negative about staying at home while our partners work, which of these things that we've talked about would have a negative effect on the relationship between you and your partner? For example, Bill, you said you don't like asking for money—how does that affect your relationship?

The discussion went on for 5 minutes and included talk about the pros and cons of being the person who brings home the paycheck.

FACILITATOR: Who benefits by all this?

JOHN: Men, sort of, but not completely.

FACILITATOR: How do men benefit?

JOHN: Well, it gives us more freedom to work outside the house, you know, more say over the money. But it also makes men into paychecks. A lot of women just see men as paychecks.

GARY: See, the whole thing is supposedly set up for men, but it backfires on them by turning them into paychecks in women's eyes.

JOHN: Yeah.

BILL: Lots of women marry men for what they can get.

FACILITATOR: I think that's true. But why is it true?

BILL: 'Cause that's how women are.

FACILITATOR: How is that, Bill? How are women?

BILL: They know how to use men. They manipulate.

FACILITATOR: Why do you think some women come to see men as paychecks?

GARY: Because men make more money. Men are supposed to be the breadwinners. Women are taught to be that way, just like men are taught to be domineering or aggressive.

FACILITATOR: So women are manipulative, taught to use men, and they're paid less than men. Is that why they think of men as paychecks?

GARY: Well, somehow it's all connected.

FACILITATOR: Before we go on can we define some of these words we're using? What does it mean to be manipulative or to manipulate?

CLAY: It means to get things set up so you get what you want—only you do it in a sneaky way.

FACILITATOR: By sneaky, does that have to be dishonest?

CLAY: No. But not up front.

FACILITATOR: You mean indirect?

CLAY: Yeah, indirect.

FACILITATOR: Do people agree with that?
(Several nodding heads.)

FACILITATOR: So we're saying that women are taught to get from men things that they want or need in indirect ways?
(More nodding heads.)

FACILITATOR: Why? Why aren't women just direct about what they want?

JACK: Because then they might not get what they want.

FACILITATOR: OK, then it seems that it also has to do with how much control women have in getting what they want. Is that right?

JACK: Yeah, if she can just get what she wants, she'd be happy.

The group then discussed the way one's ability to make decisions about one's life influences how directly one deals with other people.

The facilitator also pointed out that manipulation is tied to the system within which it is occurring. The pyramid is used as a visual representation of this. When people are operating within systems in which they do not have direct influence or power, they find ways to influence those who do. Often, what may be labeled "manipulative" is, in fact, the use of indirect influence by those without the ability to exercise direct control.

In summarizing this aspect of the discussion the facilitator pointed out that manipulation occurs in systems in which there is an imbalance of power, whether it is between parents and children, managers and workers, administrators and police officers, teachers and students, or husbands and wives.

Step 3. Relationship to the use of violence.

FACILITATOR: How does all this fit into battering? Have any of you ever hit or been abusive to your partner because you thought she was manipulating you or using you for money?
(Several men nod.)

FACILITATOR: Fred, you're nodding. What's the connection for you?

FRED: When I got arrested, it was for that.

FACILITATOR: For what?

FRED: For hitting Sheryl after a fight about leaving the bar. She didn't want to go when I wanted to, so she got into this pool match that lasted for hours. I knew she did it on purpose so I couldn't make her leave.

FACILITATOR: So you interpret that as manipulative? She wanted to stay in the bar, and instead of making her feelings known, she made it happen indirectly by getting into a pool match.

FRED: Yeah, I still think she was manipulating me.

FACILITATOR: Why didn't she just say, "Go ahead and leave, Fred. I'll get a ride with someone else"? That would have been direct.

The group went on to discuss Fred's situation and how decisions are made in their relationship. The discussion also showed that Sheryl wasn't "allowed" to stay without Fred, which meant the only way she could stay was to influence or manipulate events indirectly.

JACK: So you're saying a guy is just supposed to stay around for 2 hours and watch his old lady play pool or leave her in a bar alone?

FACILITATOR: Your what?

TIM: "Old lady" is out, Jack, you have to use her name or call her your partner or wife when you talk about her.

JACK: What's this, women's lib?

FACILITATOR: Sort of, but let's finish this and we'll come back later to this "old lady" thing.

JACK: OK, are you saying I'm supposed to just leave her there?

FACILITATOR: If you go to a bar with a male friend and he wants to stay longer than you, how would you resolve that problem? Or let me ask this—is there a problem in that case, other than the fact that you both came in one car?

JACK: It's not that simple. She isn't a guy.

FACILITATOR: But do you have a right to make her leave when you want to?

The group continued to talk about Fred's use of violence to make Sheryl leave the bar. Discussion focused on the statement "She manipulated me so I hit her" as a justification for violence and as a victim-blaming statement.

Step 4. Eliminating related violence

FACILITATOR: OK, so what are we saying? We started out saying that there is a problem when one person in a relationship works for pay and the other for free, which somehow led us to the discussion on women as manipulators. There is an important relationship between these two ideas. It's important for us to look at the root causes of problems and how a problem might be a part of a structure or a system.
(At this point the facilitator draws a pyramid on the board and shows the connections between family, structure, the economic structure of the family, and the use of indirect actions by those at the bottom of the structure to influence decisions.)

JACK: It sounds like there is nothing you can do except have both people work and make exactly the same amount of money or else this stuff goes on.

FACILITATOR: Well, it might be useful now to list some practical things that could be done in a family to get rid of or at least lessen the negative effects of one person working for pay and the other working at home for free. Bill, why don't you start? What kinds of things could you and your partner have done to make that experience of her bringing home the paycheck make you feel less dependent on her?

In this group the facilitator encouraged the participants to talk about specific ways to reduce their partners' economic dependence. This dependence may occur because they make less (or no) money or because they do not share in deciding how the money will be spent.

In summary, the exploration of a belief can take a few minutes or an hour and a half. The facilitator learns when to leave the control log to explore a belief, and when to bring that discussion back to the control log. Obviously, a group cannot explore every belief that comes up in a group. A group usually explores one or two beliefs every session.

These discussions take time—30 to 40 minutes—to reach a better understanding of violence and abusive behaviors. Again, if the group begins to think critically and reflectively, the facilitator does best to let the process go and summarize the other points on the log in five or ten minutes.

Feelings

Figure 3.6 presents the feelings section of the log.

> 3. FEELINGS: What feelings were you having?
> **Mad, frustrated**

Figure 3.6 Example of feelings section of control log.

Objectives

The group's objectives in examining the feelings section of the log follow:

1. To help participants see the connection between their beliefs and their negative feelings.
2. To help participants see the connection between the authoritarian (hierarchical) structures they cling to and the breakdown of intimate feelings and trust.
3. To help participants move beyond managing negative feelings (e.g., anger, jealousy, insecurity) to letting go of the need to control and the feelings of fear that system creates.
4. To help participants identify the wide range of their emotional responses to situations and the source of those emotions.
5. To encourage participants to experience all of their feelings, including pain, without striking out against others.
6. To help participants see that feelings such as insecurity and fear are created or exacerbated when they become abusive.

Process

Whether the group members are logging the vignette/role play or their own experiences, there are probably many feelings the group can list.

Once the group or individual has identified several feelings, the facilitator refers to the belief statements recorded in section 2. What are the connections between what a man believes and the emotions the situation brought out in him?

FACILITATOR: Jerry, you said you were insecure about Pearl wanting to go on vacation with her friends. Let's go back to your intent. You said "to make her feel guilty" and "to ruin her trip." So, all of this is going on with you—you feel left out, insecure, abandoned, and she's plowing ahead making her plans to go camping. We didn't record a belief statement for you. What would it be?

JERRY: I don't know—I guess, a couple should go on vacation together.

FACILITATOR: OK. Why? I need another one. A couple should vacation together why? (Records belief statement that "A couple is to be like one.") If you believe that being married makes you one, then every time she does something apart from you it will stir up a lot of those feelings, I assume. And where does your ability to do and go where you want enter into this?

Let's look at two things. First, the idea that we become one in marriage. Then let's look at the problem of how lousy you feel when she acts as a separate person and how that motivates you to hurt her. Anybody else here have some of these same issues?

(Several men nod.)

JERRY: Because that's what it means to be a couple.

FACILITATOR: What does it mean?

JERRY: To be like one—you know, a union.

The facilitator first asks the participants to think about how they distinguish between what "became one" when they became partners and what didn't. Obviously they don't both have to order the same food at a restaurant or go to the bathroom together. The facilitator asks a series of questions: Do you think your partner should share your taste in music? In drinks? Should she go to bed when you do? Should she share your choice of friends? Through these questions the men are challenged to examine their own rules about when their partners can be separate and when they can't.

Based on that discussion, the facilitator draws a pyramid on the board and talks about how people at the bottom of the pyramid are obligated to give up their identity and exist on some level for the people on the top. Using slavery, a colonial relationship, or an oppressively structured workplace as an example, the facilitator can draw a picture of the consciousness of domination.

In almost all discussion on feelings, it is important to put the discussion into the context of beliefs and expectations participants have of relationships with women.

In some instances the facilitator pursues the issue of expressing feelings in this discussion, but that issue is generally left for the third week, when the group discusses noncontrolling behavior.

Again, much of the theory of the curriculum is taught here.

Minimization, Denial, and Blame

Figure 3.7 presents the minimization, denial, and blame section of the log.

> 4. MINIMIZATION, DENIAL, AND BLAME: In what ways did you minimize or deny your actions or blame her?
>
> **She spit at me, that's why I had to grab her.**

Figure 3.7. Example of minimization, denial, and blame section of control log.

Objectives

The group's objectives in examining the minimization, denial, and blame section of the log follow:

1. To reinforce on a weekly basis the issue raised in the theme on accountability and honesty.
2. To help men see how blaming keeps them and anything else from changing positively.
3. To change group members' perception of being victims of the women they batter.

Process

Group members will frequently have difficulty acknowledging their responsibility for their abusive behaviors. The facilitator encourages each man to remember names he called his partner or things he said to blame her. Some men will use blaming statements when they report their actions. Often the blame is part of an internal dialogue ("self-talk") that the abuser never verbalizes to his partner.

If there are cofacilitators, the facilitator who is not at the board leading the discussion can be taking notes. A man will often blame his partner or other people when first describing the actions he used for control. The second facilitator can point out those blaming statements. Does his interpretation of the event cast him as the victim and her as the victimizer? Why? How? What does he gain from that? This issue is dealt with as part of Theme Five on accountability, but it needs to be raised in every group because it is the primary way batterers keep their system of control going. A second method of generating a group discussion on how the man in the vignette/role play or a group member blamed, minimized, or denied is demonstrated in the following exchange:

FACILITATOR: When Steve stomped out of the house he went somewhere. John, have you ever stomped out?

JOHN: Yeah, maybe once or twice.

FACILITATOR: Where did you go?

JOHN: To a bar.

FACILITATOR: So, let's say Steve took off, went to the bar and saw a friend. How did he tell his friend what happened?

PETE: He said the old lady was out tramping around all day, came prancing in at dinner time, and bitched him out for asking where she was.

JOHN: Yeah, she had an attitude, which means she must have been up to something.

FACILITATOR: Why? Why does he paint that picture to his friend?

JOHN: To get sympathy.

FACILITATOR: Sympathy? How so?

Effects

Figure 3.8 presents the effects section of the log.

5. EFFECTS: What was the impact of your action?

On you   **_spent the night in the car_**

On her   **_she's scared_**

On others   **_kids woke up crying_**

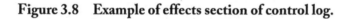

Figure 3.8   Example of effects section of control log.

Objectives

The group's objectives in examining the effects section of the log follow:

1. To motivate participants to change by helping them see the self-defeating nature of their behaviors.
2. To help the participants develop empathy for those affected by their violence and abuse.
3. To acknowledge the things participants gain by being violent and again confront the notion of themselves as victims.

Process

Showing the video *A Woman's Perspective*,[1] reading short stories by battered women, or having several formerly battered women speak to the group is helpful in generating a meaningful discussion on effects. *A Woman's Perspective* is a series of 5- to 9-minute videotaped segments drawn from a 4-hour discussion among six women, five who were battered and one who grew up in a violent home. The discussions focus on the eight tactics on the Power and Control Wheel.

During most sessions the group can simply discuss the effects of their violent and controlling behavior. At least twice during the 24-week cycle, however, it is important to focus on this segment of the log. By working with the shelter or an advocacy group, programs will have access to films or panels of women for these discussions.

It is important to ask the participants to be clear about who is affected by their behavior. For example, when a man is asked, "How did it affect you?" he may respond, "She was angry." The facilitator follows up by asking, "How does your wife being angry affect you?" In exploring what a man has gained from his action, it is useful to refer back to his intents—did she stop talking, did she stay home, was she scared, and did he get more power? The group members will often not volunteer what they got out of their actions. Usually there is a short-term gain and a long-term loss. Often the short-term gain—she gave up a friend, for instance—is also a loss to him because she resents him for it. It is important, however, not to let men portray themselves as victims of their own violence or as hurt by the battering as the women they are abusing.

Past Violence

Figure 3.9 presents the past violence section of the log.

6. PAST VIOLENCE: How did your past use of violence affect this situation?
   Made her afraid, she went to the courts.

Figure 3.9 Example of past violence section of control log.

Objectives

The group's objectives in examining the past violence section of the log follow:

1. To keep the group aware of the ongoing impact of violence on the relationship and on the women they battered.
2. To assist participants in understanding how past abuse alters their partners' actions and freedom to express themselves.

Process

Generally this discussion is brief, but there are several points to be raised in the group when discussing the effects of a man's past use of violence:

- Continued use of controlling or abusive tactics keeps his partner in fear of a resumption of violence.
- Past use of violence makes statements such as "You'd better watch out" more powerful.

- Past use of violence may add to his feeling of guilt and her distance, and it will always affect her interpretation of his current behaviors.
- If he has apologized for hitting her in the past and is now intimidating her, she doesn't believe his apology is authentic.

Noncontrolling Behaviors

Figure 3.10 presents the noncontrolling behaviors section of the log.

7. NON-CONTROLLING BEHAVIORS: What could you have done differently?
I should have left as soon as she started yelling at me.

Figure 3.10 Example of noncontrolling behaviors section of control log.

This is the focus of week 3 of each theme.

Objectives

The group's objectives in examining the noncontrolling behaviors section of the log follows:

1. To give participants opportunities to practice nonthreatening and noncontrolling reactions to situations they normally try to control.
2. To make the ideas and theories discussed in the group concrete.

Process

The process for examining what a man could have done differently is discussed in the next section, which describes the primary methods used for teaching nonviolent, noncontrolling ways of responding to conflict. These methods are role plays, lecture, and group discussion.

Use of Role Plays

Role plays are an effective teaching tool in men's groups. They give participants an opportunity to practice noncontrolling behavior, to watch how others interact, and to experience what it feels like when controlling tactics are being used by role playing their partners.

Many facilitators are nervous about using role plays. Some of the facilitators at the DAIP have had training in doing role plays or psychodrama, and others have just plunged right in.

Judy

The first night we tried role plays I thought, "No way is this going to work. These guys are going to sit and stare at us when we suggest it—and nobody will play the part of a woman." But Ty just stood up and invited one of the men to try something out. He got this guy up to the front of the room, and he played out the whole scene he had with his wife. The group was more involved than I had seen them in months.

John

The first time I tried to get someone to do a role play in group, I was shocked at how much more I understood about what the men meant when they were describing their behavior. All of a sudden I could see in detail what Frank meant by discussing things "calmly." It opened my eyes regarding how much we need to teach and how concrete we need to be about new behaviors. When one of the men would role play a situation in which he needed to negotiate rather than dominate, it was just domination in a quiet style. These role plays really let me know how the men are using the information they get in group. They can say the words you want to hear, but they can't really act out a situation without a lot of their real attitudes coming through.

Michelle

I like to play the part of the woman in the role plays, although I know some facilitators think the other group members should always do it. But if I play the woman's part, I can guide the role play more to see how he deals with her anger or set up situations in which his partner is hostile, compliant, or fearful.

Role plays are used during the third week of exploring a theme. They are used in conjunction with various exercises to teach alternative behaviors such as time-outs, negotiating, fair fighting, expressing thoughts and feelings in a noncontrolling manner, and dealing with women's anger or fear.

Role Plays Based on Curriculum Stories

Role plays are used to teach noncontrolling ways of reacting to a situation. During week 1 of each theme, the facilitators either show a vignette or role play a story, and the group logs that situation. During week 3, in lieu of role playing a man's log, the participants can role play alternative behavior to that demonstrated in the story presented during week 1 of the theme.

The facilitator asks the participant doing the role play to experience the feelings of the man in the story. For example, if the group has viewed or acted out the story *Going to School Doesn't Make You Smart* (Chapter 5, Theme Seven), the facilitator asks the participant to assume the same feelings Steve is having (the group has identified them as insecurity, defensiveness, and anger). In the role play he discusses with whomever is role-playing Cathy her decision to go to school. He has to do this without being controlling, but while believing she'll leave him or find him less desirable or necessary if she's in school.

When the role play is complete, the participants give examples of controlling and noncontrolling behaviors that came out during the role play. The facilitators may repeat the role play several times with different volunteers. It is often very difficult for the men to feel and believe as they do and to be noncontrolling. For most of them at this point in their process of change, explaining their feelings to their partners carries with it an expectation that their partners will make them feel better. The facilitator explains to the group that the expression of feelings must not be used as a tactic to gain something or to obtain forgiveness. Group members are encouraged to find other supportive people with whom to talk about their feelings when doing so with their partners places a burden on them. If and when trust is restored in the relationship, the free expression of feelings between partners is, of course, to be encouraged.

Role Plays Based on Personal Experience

Role plays are usually based on personal experiences described on the men's logs in the previous week. The facilitator asks for a volunteer and then paraphrases what the man wrote on his log and asks some additional questions so the group gets a fairly clear sense of what transpired. He is asked to recreate the situation with another participant who will play his partner, but the volunteer is to act nonabusively rather than abusively as he recorded on his log.

If a participant is role playing one of his own experiences, he should remember and re-experience the feelings he was having. He reenacts the incident, this time practicing noncontrolling behavior.

After the role play, the facilitators ask for feedback from the group. Was he still being controlling or abusive?

Some facilitators videotape the scenes so participants can see and hear how they react to conflict.

The following are a few ground rules to set for role plays:

- There should not be any physical contact between the two people role playing a situation.
- The participants can stop the role play at any time.

- The facilitators should give a clear explanation of what the goal of the role play is.
- Before the role play begins, the facilitator should try to outline as clearly as possible what transpired in the situation to be role played by asking the participants questions. What was your tone of voice? How close to her were you when you were arguing? What exact words did you use? (It is not so important, however, to replay the words and gestures as the power dynamics and feelings.)
- The female cofacilitator should not be put in the position of role playing the female part, unless she feels comfortable doing this. It can be extremely useful to have the men role playing the partner's role.
- If the role play gets off track, the facilitators can stop the role play and ask specific questions to get it back on track by either referring to the log or the story.
- After getting feedback from the group, ask both people how they felt in their roles.

After doing several role plays, the facilitators choose a skill-building exercise that relates to the basic issues that come out of the discussion. The exercises provide an opportunity for the facilitators to help men change entrenched patterns of behavior.

Other exercises

The following exercises provide several skill-building techniques:

1. Time-outs: Perhaps the most widely used skill-building technique in counseling and educational programs for abusers is the "time-out" exercise. The concept, adapted from Dr. Anne Ganley's work, involves teaching the participant to recognize when he is at the point at which he may become abusive and then to leave the situation until his anger subsides. This skill is taught at the orientation session and should be discussed throughout the men's participation in groups.

The appropriate use of a time-out occurs when conflict escalates to the point at which an individual believes he will become abusive if he stays in that situation. The facilitator may wish to show the vignette or role play both versions of the story *You're Not Going Bowling* to illustrate the practice of time-outs. The role play for Version One is described in Chapter 5, Theme One. In it, Curtis demands to know where Jackie's going and tells her she can't leave. When she tries to go anyway, he taunts and then hits her. In Version Two, Curtis takes a time out. In doing so, he does several positive things, but also does several things that could leave Jackie in fear of further abuse.

Your're Not Going Bowling (Version Two)

It's Jackie's bowling night and she's getting ready to go out. Curtis confronts Jackie about her going bowling. Jackie tells Curtis that he goes out drinking with his friends so she is entitled to go bowling with her friends. Curtis gets angry, towers over her, and says, "That's another thing, your friends. I don't like your friends—they're are a bunch of . . ." Curtis stops talking and says that he has to leave, although he doesn't say he is taking a time-out. He leaves.

Jackie returns from bowling. Curtis is sitting reading a magazine. He asks Jackie if they can talk. Jackie is a little cool but sits down. Curtis apologizes for his behavior and tells Jackie that he gets jealous of her. Jackie asks, "Do you want me to stay home every night, is that what you want?" Curtis acknowledges that she needs her own life and that he took a long walk and thought about things and that he will change. He also says that he called his group leader, and he will bring up what happened at group tomorrow. He again apologizes. He is very calm and remains seated throughout the discussion.

Exercise on time-outs

Divide the chalkboard or flipchart into two columns headed "Positive Aspects" and "Negative Aspects." After showing or role playing Versions One and Two of *You're Not Going Bowling*, the facilitator asks the group to list the positive and negative aspects of Curtis's time-out. The facilitator then leads a discussion on one's responsibilities when taking time-outs. A sample follows:

POSITIVE ASPECTS	NEGATIVE ASPECTS
• Doesn't use violence. • Leaves the house. • Takes a walk. • Calls his group leader or group member. • Doesn't blame her. • Apologizes. • Says he will bring it up in group.	• Doesn't leave before he becomes abusive. • Doesn't say he is taking a time-out. • Doesn't say where he is going. • Doesn't say when he is coming back.

During the discussion, the facilitator points out the need for participants to follow specific rules and agreements they have made with their partners when they feel they may be getting abusive.

In Version Two, even though Curtis doesn't use physical violence, he does tell Jackie he doesn't want her to go and towers over her in a very threatening manner. When Curtis doesn't say where he is going or when he is coming back, Jackie doesn't know what to expect when he returns. He may have become more agitated or gotten drunk, or he may not come home at all.

After discussing the exercise, it may be helpful to reiterate time-out rules. The following guidelines for taking a time-out are recommended:

- Use time-outs when you believe you are about to become abusive. Do not use them to avoid conflict or disagreement.
- State that you are taking a time-out, don't just leave.

- Use positive self-talk and other relaxation techniques during your time-outs.
- Do not use drugs or alcohol during your time-out.
- Get positive support from other group members, friends, or family.
- Call before you return. Ask if she feels safe, and honor her request to stay away if she feels unsafe.
- Do not insist on dealing with the conflict immediately on returning.

For responsible time-outs to occur, it's important that the partners of participants know the rules of time-outs. Without a thorough explanation, time-outs can be controlling and sometimes dangerous. The time-out exercise can be explained to the partners of participants by shelter advocates or at women's orientation sessions.

2. **Acknowledgment of women's fear:** Almost all of the men participating in the DAIP groups have ongoing contact with their partners. About half of them are living with the women they battered. Frequently men will make comments such as the following:

- "She's using this court thing to get even."
- "She keeps throwing this 'You're a batterer' crap in my face."
- "I don't think she's scared anymore. She knows I'm not going to hit her."
- "She's got the shelter, the courts, everybody on her side. It's not fair."

If these statements are getting nods of approval from the other group members, the facilitator might ask "How many of you think your partner is still afraid of you?" or "How long do you think it takes for someone not to be afraid after being physically assaulted?" or "Why wouldn't she be afraid that it would happen again?"

Exercise on acknowledging women's fear

Show the vignette *You Act Like You've Already Got the Money Spent* or role play a story in which a man threatens his partner verbally and then immediately starts to apologize, saying he didn't mean it.

You Act Like You've Already Got The Money Spent

Kay is preparing a meal for Blake in the kitchen when a discussion begins about when the tax return check will come. Blake tells Kay that he is anxious about the check coming, and Kay says that she has been checking the mail every day. Blake gets angry and accuses Kay of already having the money spent. He states that when the check comes, he wants it all to go to the car because he won't be able to work without transportation. Kay becomes angry at his overreaction and tells him, "The car doesn't work because you and your friends beat the car to death and if you would grow up . . ." Blake becomes enraged, gets up from the table and screams, "Look, bitch, shut the fuck up." He is only a few inches from Kay, who is clearly afraid. Blake apologizes and says he just "lost it."

This scene may be very familiar to men who have recently stopped physically assaulting their partners because of a court order or an arrest. Many of the group members are afraid of jail, so they aren't hitting their partners, but they are still using threats and intimidation. This discussion should focus on three questions.

Question 1:   What happens when men stop hitting because of the threat of jail?

For those men who are still living with their partners, the impact of the arrest or protection order and the threat of jail is immediate. Below is an example of a discussion after watching this film.

FACILITATOR: What changed for you, Bill, after you were put on probation?

BILL: It seems like she can say anything she wants to now because she knows if I get mad, I'll end up in jail.

FRANK: Yeah, they know when they've got you over a barrel.

FACILITATOR: What do you mean by "over a barrel"?

BILL: You know, she knows that the guy can go to jail. The wife says to me—

FACILITATOR: Who?

(Laughter. There is a rule in the group that the men have to refer to their partners by name.)

BILL: Sandy. So anyway, Sandy says to me, "If you ever touch me, I'll call the cops, and you'll go to jail." She uses it as a threat.

FACILITATOR: How is that a threat? She's telling you that if you assault her, she'll call the police, and you will end up in jail. That doesn't sound like a threat, but a commitment to doing whatever she can to protect herself from getting hit again.

BILL: Well, yeah, but it's the tone of voice and all that. She uses it to get me. She knows I'm not going to hit her.

FACILITATOR: How does she know that?

BILL: She knows it.

FACILITATOR: Have you ever stopped hitting her in the past and said it'll never happen again? (No answer.)

FACILITATOR: Didn't you go to counseling a couple years ago and then say you wouldn't hit her?

BILL: Yeah, I guess.

FACILITATOR: So I'd guess that it'll take her more than a promise to believe that you won't hit her again.

The group went on to discuss the issue of violence as a tactic of control and the ongoing effects of violence on women's lives.

Bill's statement that Sandy can say anything she wants to, presumably because he can't hit her anymore, allows the facilitator to show how Bill's violence was used to control Sandy and to challenge Bill's perception that he is a victim. Many men intellectually grasp and even agree with the argument that their use of violence has been to control their partners' actions, thoughts, and feelings, but they need to internalize what that means. Bill's opening statement (paraphrased), "I can't hit her, so now she is free to talk," needs to be explored. If Bill can truly understand the implications of that statement, he will start to see how he is minimizing and denying his abuse and setting himself up as her victim. He then has the choice to continue to blame her or to accept responsibility for his behavior and its intent. Bill had always been able to stop Sandy from talking before and now that he can't hit her, he can't stop her.

Following is an example of how to explore this:

FACILITATOR: Bill, I'm going to restate your opening remark and then I have some questions for you. (Facilitator writes on board.) "I can't hit her anymore—so now she can say whatever she wants." Is that an accurate way of writing what your statement meant?

BILL: That's it. Doesn't sound good though.

FACILITATOR: It sounds real. It's more clear when written like this on the board. So now what, Bill—what do you think is going to happen if you can't stop Sandy from talking by hitting her?

BILL: She'll probably get away with murder.

FACILITATOR: You mean she'll be verbally abusive to you now.

BILL: Yeah, she is.

FACILITATOR: So now you can't hit her anymore, now what are you going to do?

BILL: I don't know. Find some other way of shutting her up I guess, or just walk out.

FACILITATOR: How about in the film? How did Blake shut Kay up?

BILL: He went at her like he was going to hit her.

FACILITATOR: So Kay in this scene was saying whatever she wanted even though Blake didn't like it. Is that what you're saying Sandy is doing now?

BILL: Yeah, but worse.

FACILITATOR: Okay. Let's stick with Blake for a minute. Why did he do what he did?

BILL: Because she was blaming him for the car needing to be fixed. He wanted her to shut up.

FACILITATOR: Did he have the right to do what he did?

BILL: What do you mean by "the right"?

FACILITATOR: You know, like rights that we all believe we have, like I have the right to voice my opinion or the right to tell my side of the story. You know, like what is fair. Was it fair what he did?

BILL: Well no, I guess it wasn't fair.

FACILITATOR: Why wasn't it fair?

BILL: Because she's smaller than him so he can just bully her into shutting up.

This discussion concluded with Bill's acknowledgment that his statement made him sound like a victim when in fact he wasn't.

Question 2: Why wouldn't a woman who was assaulted or threatened accept an apology?

This is an important issue when talking to men about abuse. Many of the participants won't allow their partners to be angry about their past use of violence and refuse to accept the ongoing consequences of their use of violence.

FACILITATOR: Has anyone here had this happen? Have you apologized, and she won't accept it or doesn't want to hear it?

FRANK: Sure, lots of times. It's like she won't forget.

The facilitator then discusses the following with the group:

- Why aren't women able to forget past use of violence?
- How does it feel to have your partner afraid of you? (Long-term consequences of battering.)
- What needs to happen to have a woman feel safe after she has been hit or when she lives with a man she knows has battered another woman?

Question 3: In the vignette/role play has Blake made the decision to stop battering?

Many participants find this question difficult to discuss because they don't perceive their behavior as battering unless they use physical violence.

SAM: I don't know if he'll never do it, but I think he was sincere that he didn't want to hit her again.

JACK: If he was sincere, he wouldn't have gone after her like that.

SAM: I think he didn't want to hit her—if he did he would have.

JACK: Maybe, but he still wants her to shut up when he doesn't want to hear what she's saying.

The facilitator then leads the discussion to these points:

- A man can't just stop hitting. He also has to stop forcing his will on his partner.
- Shifting from physical abuse to another form of abuse does not stop battering. The battering continues, but now it's legal.

This discussion can be tied into Theme Five on accountability as the acknowledgment of one's actions and the acceptance of responsibility for them.

3. Acceptance of women's anger: The anger of people who are dominated by another is always powerful. Whites are afraid of the anger of people of color, parents are afraid of their teenagers' anger, management is afraid of labor's anger and men are afraid of women's anger. Women's anger reveals to men their outrage, resentment, resistance, and defiance. Anger is also a feeling that women are discouraged from showing, whereas it is often the only feeling that men are encouraged to express.

There are different ways all of us, especially abusers, block another person's anger. One effective method is simply to say, "I don't know what you're talking about, I don't understand." A second way is to accuse the angry person of attacking. A third way is to attack the person who is getting angry: "What about when you . . . ?" A fourth way, which many men use to respond to women's anger, is to trivialize it, to laugh at them when they get angry. In one segment in the video *A Woman's Perspective*, a woman talks about her husband's response to her anger. He put his hand on her head and held her at arm's length, as if she was threatening to him, and then laughed at her while she yelled at him. For batterers, a final way to stop anger is to use intimidation, escalating it until his partner stops, and if necessary, to stop her physically from being angry: to hit her, to put his hand over her mouth, to choke her, to force her to stop showing her anger. When a batterer explains that he couldn't take his partner's "nagging" anymore, and broke or threw something, he may in fact be describing how he stopped her expression of anger.

In this exercise participants are asked to identify how both society and they as individuals tell women not to be angry. The group examines this message's destructive effect on women, and what happens to this repressed anger. Participants then discuss what they think will happen if women are allowed to get angry, and how men and women could benefit if society and individuals within it stopped blocking women's anger.

Exercise on accepting women's anger:

A nonthreatening way of beginning this discussion is for the facilitator to ask the participants to talk about their experiences with women's anger outside of their intimate relationships. For example:

- Why do we trivialize women's anger?
- How does the media treat women's anger?
- How did your father respond to your mother's anger?
- How did you as a child respond to your mother's anger?
- How frequently have you seen movies in which people like John Wayne respond to an angry woman, "You're so beautiful when you're angry"? Or in which a man hits a woman who is yelling and screaming because she is hysterical?
- What does the word "hysterical" mean? (Frequently a woman simultaneously expressing feelings of anger and hurt is labeled hysterical.)
- What are some of the expressions we use in our society to describe women who are angry? (For example, "She's on the rag" or "It's that time of the month." Angry women are also referred to as "bitches.")

If women aren't considered important, then neither is their anger; if anger is powerful, then women shouldn't be angry, because women shouldn't be powerful. Women are to be subservient, but their anger implies that they have power, and it should therefore be stopped.

Next the facilitator can use an exercise in which participants list tactics they have used in an intimate relationship to block their partner's anger. The following are some examples.

- Walking out.
- "I don't know what you're talking about."
- "You deserve better—you should leave me."
- "I'm a horrible person. I'm no good. You're right."
- "You are even worse than me. How about when you . . ."
- Making fun of her: "So what's the big deal?" "Are you on the rag?" "You're so cute when you're mad."
- Stopping her physically, putting a hand over her mouth, intimidating her, hitting her.

After group members give examples of ways in which anger is stopped, and specifically ways in which they have stopped their partners' anger, then the question is why? Why do they stop it? What would happen if they didn't stop it? How does keeping women from being angry keep men powerful, or women powerless? How frequently is the use of violence a way to shut down women's anger? What would be different in the men's relationships with their partners if, when their partners were angry, they responded in a respectful way? When a woman gets angry and it is blocked in one of the ways listed, what happens to that anger? What is the effect on her, on him, and on the relationship when that anger is blocked?

The facilitator can easily keep the discussion going by asking any combination of these questions, but it is important to seek more than a simple response to the question. For example, "Why do we trivialize women's anger?" is a very important question, and the tendency in the group might be to treat the question lightly (which is itself a form of trivializing women's anger). Because even nonabusive men block women's anger, male facilitators may find themselves strongly empathizing with the men in the group on this issue.

Discussion should focus on how a woman's anger is an expression of herself and of her desire to influence a situation, and how a man's rejection or blocking of that anger can be an attempt to control the situation. This exercise should end by asking the group members to think about ways to listen to and nonabusively respond to women's anger.

Other exercises[2] not included in this book that are commonly used in batterer's groups are

1. Recognizing anger cues
2. Using positive self-talk
3. Using assertive behavior
4. Being aware of nonverbal cues
5. Communicating feelings and thoughts
6. Letting go
7. Fighting fairly

Helping men to develop specific skills is an important but secondary goal of this curriculum, the primary goal of which is to stop battering by challenging the belief system underlying men's violent behavior. Skill-building techniques should be used whenever an opportunity presents itself. The third week of every theme is specifically designed to explore noncontrolling behavior through the use of role plays and, when appropriate, skill-building exercises.

CONCLUSION

Many practitioners using this curriculum initially find this structure restrictive. The way the videos and exercises (particularly the control log) preclude discussion about the dynamics of a particular relationship can be frustrating.

During the past several years we have received a tremendous amount of feedback on these design decisions. Practitioners who, like us, were making the shift from a family systems approach or an anger management approach have consistently told us that the curriculum gets to the core of the issue of violence in a way that their previous approaches had not. However, many found it was difficult at first to use the logs and the role plays because they were not comfortable with where they would take the group.

This seemed to be a contradiction. On one hand the design seemed too structured and on the other hand it seemed to lead to discussions and issues that many were not comfortable exploring. Our intention has been to structurally exclude the irrelevant, which leaves the fundamental issues of power and violence and the desire for control. When we first started writing the curriculum, we asked ourselves, "What do the women who have lived through the nightmare of being battered want us to do in these groups?" This curriculum answered part of that question. Ultimately, she must decide whether his change process is a temporary response or a commitment to altering attitudes and behaviors that are destructive to her.

NOTES

1. This book, *Education Groups for Men Who Batter,* replaces our original curriculum manual, *Power & Control: Tactics of Men Who Batter.*

    Up to now, our curriculum package has been available only to those who attend training sponsored by the DAIP's National Training Project. (The package consists of this book, 13 video vignettes, the videos *A Woman's Perspective* and *Using the Control Log,* lesson plans for each of the eight themes, and posters of the Power and Control and Equality Wheels). The training teaches the use of the curriculum and focuses on the importance of batterers' programs working with women's shelters and the courts. By limiting access to the curriculum package to those who have attended training, we seek to maintain basic standards of accountability for programs using our materials.

    In publishing this work, we share the Duluth model with the increasing number of individual practitioners and community programs intervening with men who batter. In keeping with our policy on the sale of the curriculum package, the aforementioned videos and lesson plans are available only to those who attend training. For information and training, contact the National Training Project, 206 West Fourth street, Duluth, MN 55806.

2. These exercises are explained in the lesson plans for this curriculum. See above note.

Chapter 4

Role of the Facilitator

Group facilitators assume six roles.

1. To participate in an interagency effort to hold participants in a group accountable for further acts of violence and for failure to complete the rehabilitation program
2. To keep the group focused on the issues of violence, abuse, control, and change
3. To facilitate reflective and critical thinking
4. To maintain an atmosphere that is compassionate and challenging and not colluding
5. To provide new information and teach noncontrolling relationship skills
6. To facilitate a healthy group process

ROLE 1: TO PARTICIPATE IN AN INTERAGENCY EFFORT TO HOLD PARTICIPANTS IN A GROUP ACCOUNTABLE FOR FURTHER ACTS OF VIOLENCE AND FOR FAILURE TO COMPLETE THE REHABILITATION PROGRAM

The DAIP is structured so that as each man walks into his first group session he does so fully aware of the consequences of renewed violence. He does so knowing that the facilitator is working in conjunction with the officer who arrested him, the judge who sentenced him, the probation officer who supervises him, and the DAIP staff members who monitor his attendance and his ongoing use of violence.

The facilitator plays a key role in making an interagency system work. However, the facilitator, more than anyone else in the system, is vulnerable to acts of collusion with men in his or her group. Making the decision to report all acts of violence, to warn women of threats, or to refuse to write a letter to the court on a client's behalf can be difficult, as the following facilitator discovered.

Steven

I was all in favor of police officers losing discretion and being forced to arrest in cases in which they had the evidence. But about six or seven weeks into my first group, a guy that I had really come to admire slapped his wife. It was one of those really ugly fights, and she said some things to him that just went to the gut. I understood how frustrated he was. He was honest about it, he knew it was wrong, and I just did not want to report him to his probation officer. But his conditions of probation were clear: "No violence." It didn't say, "No violence unless she says something really ugly." So I waited. Two facilitators' meetings went by and finally I reported him. Actually, I mentioned it in passing and, of course, quite a few people picked up on the fact that I was supposed to report it. I mumbled about being unsure of the rule if he self-reported, but I knew the policy. He ended up getting a weekend in jail and starting group over. Looking back, it was probably the best thing to happen to him and to her, but at the time I got caught up in how good he was doing. I think the only way to handle these situations now is through team discussion. Making these decisions alone is just not a wise thing.

The following are excerpts from the DAIP counseling agency agreement that defines the role of each facilitator in the intervention process:

- The DAIP staff will update facilitators and counselors on changes in probationary status, orders for protection, and reports of additional acts of violence committed by participants in their groups. However, such information from a victim will not be used without her permission. (In many cases facilitators or counselors are aware of new acts of violence committed by a group member, but they do not confront him because this would further threaten the victim's safety.)

- Facilitators and counselors will report all new acts of violence committed by a participant to the men's program coordinator at the DAIP and discuss appropriate actions by the program. The women's program coordinator or the facilitator or counselor will contact the victim to determine the nature of the new offense, injuries, details of the incident, and a description of what else is going on in the relationship (e.g., intimidating behavior, psychological control, and the implications to the victim if the court is informed of the new offense). An act of violence will result in a consequence (e.g., revocation of probation, imposition of some jail time and starting the program over, civil court action, or required attendance at an additional number of sessions). An individual who commits a repeat offense will be told that his or her involvement at the DAIP is on a probationary status. Participants will remain in group until the criminal or civil court has determined the consequence for the repeat offense. If the women's program coordinator, the counselor, or the victim believes that reporting acts of violence to the court will place the victim in danger, the matter will be discussed at the next team meeting. The team will provide input to the DAIP staff on an appropriate recommendation to the probation officer.

- Counselors will report to the DAIP weekly on attendance at group sessions.
- Counselors will report any alleged incidents of child abuse to an initial intervention unit or child protection worker from social services.
- Representatives of the counseling agencies participating in the DAIP will attend the bimonthly team meetings with the DAIP staff and education group facilitators, a representative from the probation department, and other participants in the program to promote interagency communication and conduct continued evaluation of the counseling and educational groups.

ROLE 2: TO KEEP THE GROUP FOCUSED ON THE ISSUES OF VIOLENCE, ABUSE, CONTROL, AND CHANGE

Men who physically attack their partners are carrying out a destructive behavior pattern that extends beyond their individual acts of violence. It doesn't take long for a facilitator to get tangled up in all of the issues men bring up in the groups including alcoholism, family histories of violence, poor communication skills, inability to identify or express feelings, "short fuses," poor self-images, unemployment, and feelings of being victimized by their partners and the world around them.

This curriculum is based on the premise that the purpose of using physical abuse in relationships is to control the thoughts, feelings, or actions of another person. The following excerpt from a transcript of a men's group demonstrates the way a facilitator focused on the issue of control.

FACILITATOR: Bob, you're saying that you wouldn't "let" your wife go to work because that was your job. What do you mean by "let her work?" Is working outside the home your job only?

BOB: Well, that's how I grew up. My dad worked and my mom stayed home. If a guy can't support his family, I've always thought there was something wrong with him.

MARK: Don't you think all of us grew up doing what our fathers did? Don't you think it works both ways? Women grew up thinking that way too.

FACILITATOR: I just don't think these things happen out of the blue. Why is it set up like that? That men go out and work, and women work in the home without pay?

PETE: It's that way in order to keep order.

FACILITATOR: Order?

PETE: Well, some roles have to be set in order to keep things from falling apart.

FACILITATOR: But if men's work or role is to make money and women's work or role is without pay, what does that do?

PETE: It makes women dependent on men for money—but you have to remember that it also uses men, she owes it to him to take care of the home because he's busting his ass all day.

FACILITATOR: What does it mean in the family that he brings home the paycheck?

JOHN: He gets to make the decisions, he's paid for that.

FACILITATOR: What do men get out of it being set up that way?

PETE: We get old fast and have heart attacks at 50.

JOHN: We get to make family decisions.

FACILITATOR: So Bob, when you say you wouldn't let your wife go out and work, what were you going to get out of that? Why wouldn't you want all that money coming in?

BOB: Not for power if that's what you're saying.
(Several men laugh.)

FACILITATOR: I never mentioned power. You did.

BOB: Yeah, but you're always bringing up power.

FACILITATOR: OK, we have listed on the board 20 ways that men in the group have imposed their decisions on their partners, and you're saying one way you do it is by not letting her work. When you look at this list, for example, "not letting her see certain friends," "not letting her go to school," "not letting her take a vacation alone," don't you think it has something to do with power?

BOB: I suppose it does when you look at it that way, but I don't know if each of us individually thinks of it as getting power when we do it.

FACILITATOR: OK, in your individual case, why did you keep your wife from working?

BOB: Because she didn't need to work.

MARK: Was she independently wealthy?

BOB: No, I was working.

As the facilitator pursued this with the group, Bob finally came up with the following statement:

BOB: If she's working, she won't need me.

FACILITATOR: She won't need you for money, then will she leave you?

BOB: Yeah, maybe.

FACILITATOR: Why would she leave you? What besides money does she get in her relationship with you?

BOB: Not much, I guess.

FACILITATOR: It sounds like keeping her financially dependent also lets you not care much about how you treat her.

(Bob makes no response.)

JOHN: That's how it was with my wife and when the kids moved out, she did too. She just walked out. She'd just had enough, I guess.

A man's violence against his partner is inextricably linked to his perception of the world and her place in it. Without a change in his world view, the violent man will continue to find "legitimate" reasons to impose his will on his partner physically.

Human beings are products of their world but are also able to act to change their world. The men in the groups will often talk about their violence as a response to being victimized. They see themselves as victims: victims of a violent childhood; victims of an economy in which there is no place for them; victims of a society that makes them hide their feelings; victims of a court system that doesn't care why an incident happened, only that it happened; victims of a culture that tells them to be in control even when they don't want to be; victims of a culture that separates men from their children; victims of women who won't follow the rules; and victims of women who won't make it all better.

The reality is that many batterers have been abused in the past and now feel victimized by their partners. A man like this will rarely end his violence without changing the way he views his relationship. His thinking has many contradictions. The facilitator helps focus his thinking on the choice to act abusively: its intent, its place in his value system, and its impact on his life.

The facilitators can provide a way for men to examine their values and goals concerning their intimate relationships with women. The group helps them look at their behaviors, not as out of control, but as the means to get or keep something. It challenges men to explore the relationship of their values to their behaviors. It inevitably also challenges the facilitator, male or female, to explore the same issues as it becomes more and more difficult to deny the use of many of the same abusive tactics and controlling behaviors with past or present partners.

ROLE 3: TO FACILITATE REFLECTIVE AND CRITICAL THINKING IN THE GROUP

Throughout this curriculum are directions such as "Lead a discussion on . . ." or "Have the group discuss . . ." or "Examine the aspects of . . ." Sometimes this sounds easier than it is. In Duluth, more than 90% of the men sitting in the room are court mandated. They don't like coming to group.

They resent the program, the courts that require them to attend, the facilitators, the women they battered. They are, however, very capable of reflective and critical thinking.

Fortunately, during the group process some men make the switch. They begin to look forward to coming to group—after all, it's the only place they can honestly talk about what's going on in their lives without all the bravado, the feigned disinterest in their relationships, the "read-my-lips" attitude.

Understanding of Culture

The analysis of critical thinking that underlies this curriculum is based on the work of Brazilian educator Paulo Freire. Critical thinking is reflective—it is critical as opposed to mystical. We live in a society that uses myth to maintain societal order in what is essentially a dysfunctional culture.

To see the world and our culture from a critical mind, we must first separate what is nature—those things made in creation (for some, by the Creator) from what is culture—those things made by humankind. Mystical thinking occurs when people believe that what are cultural phenomena are nature's way. For example, hierarchy as a social order is a cultural pattern. Its shape is the pyramid. The belief in hierarchy as a natural structure is firmly held by many men in the groups, who make statements such as "That's nature, men are men and women are women" and "The buck has to stop someplace."

The first step then in helping men think critically is to challenge mystical thinking. When a man says, "That's just the way men and women are made," "It's always been that way," or makes any other statement that suggests a cultural phenomenon to be nature's way, the facilitator asks why, how, and who made things this way? This questioning is crucial to a participant's being able or willing to change because if he can justify his behavior as in accord with "God's plan," then why should he change it?

The following are excerpts from an intake interview with a man court mandated to the groups through a civil protection order for handcuffing his wife to the bed and forcing her to have oral sex with him.

DAN: I didn't know she hated it. I mean I thought we had an agreement to act out each other's fantasies. I didn't know until the next day when she called from the shelter that she hated it.

INTAKE PERSON: What do you think influences your fantasies? Do you read men's magazines or watch movies with that kind of stuff?

DAN: No, I've seen a few but not lately.
(Dan's wife reported that he watched hard-core pornography and snuff films on his VCR several times a week and that she had erased four or five of his films the morning he raped her.)

INTAKE PERSON: I'm trying to get at what you think makes you want to dominate your wife that

> way. I imagine it was a humiliating experience for her. I think that, as men, we
> often get some sense of power out of humiliating a woman. Is that true for you?
>
> DAN: It's the nature of the beast.

The facilitator must challenge the concept that it is in men's nature to be rapists.

Stepping-Back Process

A second element in facilitating critical thinking is the stepping-back process. The curriculum uses 13 stories that are either acted out by the facilitators or presented on the videotapes which complement this series. (See note at end of Chapter 3.) These 13 stories mirror the group members' actions without producing the guilt and defensiveness that prevents them from examining their own behavior. The facilitator can also help men step back by using analogies, which removes the emotional charge accompanying discussion of personal situations. In the following example, a group member claims that his wife makes a "big deal" about his becoming upset, but that when she herself, the children, his mother-in-law, or anyone else gets angry, she overlooks it. (He was referring to throwing things and yelling as "becoming upset.")

> FACILITATOR: Dan, can we switch gears here and talk about your work? If your boss comes into the shop and starts shouting at someone and throwing things around, how would that be different from when the secretary did it?
>
> DAN: It'd be very different.
>
> FACILITATOR: How?
>
> DAN: Well, for one thing . . .

Problem Posing

The third aspect of critical thinking is problem posing. In two out of every three sessions the groups use a control log to guide the discussion. The facilitator poses a question or problem, and then keeps the group moving toward the deepest level of understanding possible at that time.

While this curriculum is purposely structured to limit the agenda to why these men batter, how they batter and how they can change, the use of the control log is enhanced by discussion that is truly dialogical. To move a discussion from list making to deeper levels of discussion, the facilitator must truly want to understand, to enter into dialogue with the group members. If the facilitator has a predetermined "correct" answer, the participants will quickly learn how to fill in the blanks of the logs and answer the question "correctly."

The following is an example of a facilitator posing questions and looking for a way to help the group members think through their beliefs.

FACILITATOR: Harold, you just spoke about how your partner "pushes your buttons." That expression is used a lot in group. What does it mean to you?

HAROLD: You know. She makes me mad.

FACILITATOR: Is that what it means for others?

WARREN: That, and she knows how to make you mad. She knows just the right thing to say or do that will get you.

HAROLD: Yeah. It's like part of getting to know someone. You know where their weaknesses are so you go for that.

FACILITATOR: I've never heard that expression in a women's group. I have heard women say that men find their weaknesses, but this button business seems to be a man's expression. Harold, do you think of your feelings in that way? They are there all the time, and if someone pushes a button, wham, out they'll come?

HAROLD: Well, sort of, I guess.

FACILITATOR: Are those feelings always there? Could I push your button by saying something?

HAROLD: Probably, but you wouldn't know you did it.

FACILITATOR: You mean you wouldn't blow up.

HAROLD: Yeah. I'd control it.

FACILITATOR: Why do you blow up with Nancy?

HAROLD: Because she's supposed to be my—no, because she does it to hurt me, to get me to blow up. If you did it, it would be kind of like an accident. You just happened upon something, and I'd brush it off.

FACILITATOR: That makes living with you sound like living in a mine field. If you step here—bang, there's an explosion. Do you think it's scary to live with you?

HAROLD: Yeah. I guess so.

FACILITATOR: How about you, Louis? Is it scary sometimes living with you?

LOUIS: Lisa says it is. So, I guess it is.

FACILITATOR: John, is it scary to live with you?

JOHN: Sometimes.

FACILITATOR: Let's spend a few minutes talking about how it got that way. John, what's one of the things that made you scary? How did it happen?

JOHN: My old man I guess. He scared the piss out of everybody. I guess I took after him.

After a discussion of the many forces that influenced the men to become intimidating the following question was posed.

FACILITATOR: What is this list? Fathers, Vietnam, the army, mothers, booze, drugs, unfaithful wives? These could all look like pretty good reasons to be violent, but how about all the men who've had those same experiences and didn't become violent—what happened with them?

The group then discussed change and the resistance we all have to it.

The facilitator steers the discussion away from victim-blaming statements about women intentionally pushing men's buttons to why the men harbor so much explosive anger and what they want to do about it. This transcript also demonstrates that in this structured curriculum, the facilitator allows the discussion to flow within boundaries and brings it back to the relationship of violence to control and the need for the men to change.

"The End Is the Means in Process"

To teach men to think critically a critical process must be created. It must be true dialogue, not simply a pitting of the facilitators against the men in a 26-week debate. Group members need to experience a process in which there doesn't always have to be a winner, as the following quote from a facilitator attests.

Wendy

> I used to go into group ready for anything they would throw at me. Most nights one of the men would make some really terrible remark about women—sometimes, I think, just for my benefit. So, I'd get into it with him. Nine times out of 10—or more—I'd win the debate. I'd go home thinking to myself that I kept the lid on that junk that night. Finally, I realized the men were winning, not me. Week after week I was doing exactly what they do at home, winning the debate.

The most important aspect of role modeling is the way the facilitator chooses to engage or not engage with men who are in essence attempting to change the purpose of the group. The facilitator's job is not to make the men "get it" or to make them change. The role is to engage them in an honest dialogue, to teach them what you know and how you came to know it, to explore with them things you do not yet know, and to work with others to hold the men accountable to the women they've abused.

The facilitator must make a commitment to seek the truth, understand the complexities of this issue, and remain inquisitive and searching. The key to this aspect of facilitating critical thinking is walking the fine line between affirmation-support and collusion-reinforcement.

The following is an example of collusion on the part of the facilitator:

> LARRY: I'm always pissed at her. She's tried to bring me down, she's taken my kids, she's taken my house, she's even got my dog. Yeah, I'm mad, and I'm always to blame.
>
> FACILITATOR: You buy into it, Larry. It's like she throws out a line, and you grab it. You take the bait and get hooked.
>
> LARRY: Yeah, I'm in there all right. I fall for her shit.

This is a common form of collusion in a men's group. Although the intent is to show Larry that he has choices, the facilitator has, in this case, reinforced Larry's claim of being a victim.

Framework for Understanding

Again and again, the facilitator translates the group discussion to the board by drawing the pyramid, moving the discussion from the context of "his relationship with her" to other hierarchical relationships in which the tactics on the Power and Control Wheel are used to maintain the system. How does the person at the top

- think?
- act?
- feel?

How does the person at the bottom

- think?
- act?
- feel?

The following are questions that help facilitate critical thinking about the relationship of authoritarian structures (economic, social, and political) to human behavior.

- Why don't the people at the bottom communicate directly with those at the top?
- What is the basis for people being at the top?
  - in the workplace?
  - in the church?
  - in the family?
  - in government?
- Why are people at the top fearful? How do they express that fear?
- Why are people at the bottom fearful? How do they express that fear?
- Are people at the top insecure?
- How would you define the insecurity of people at the top compared with the insecurity of those at the bottom?
- What is the relationship between the Power and Control Wheel and the tactics used by others in society to stay at the top?
- How do people at the bottom resist control by people at the top?

The hierarchy illustrated by the pyramid requires that one person be in control. It does not allow for an egalitarian relationship. Even though in many ways the people at the bottom submit to this structure as natural or "God's plan," or simply give up struggling, it is an unnatural state, and thus women will resent the structure and all of its implications.

To maintain the pyramid structure, a batterer must use the tactics on the Power and Control Wheel—tactics learned in the culture from birth—and must punish his partner's acts of resistance. A man becomes trapped by this system, fearing that ending his role in it will reverse the structure, and he will then be controlled by her. Because the pyramid is natural to him, he sees his position as either on the top or the bottom.

Being on the bottom does not make women naturally good. In fact, it takes a very heavy physical, emotional, intellectual, and spiritual toll on women. However, how women behave is not a causal factor in whether or not their partners are violent. This is not to say that individual acts by women don't provide the excuse or rationalization for a specific assault. It is not necessary to defend every action of a woman to avoid victim blaming. Some behavior by the women the men are abusing is quite awful, but that is irrelevant to his change process and to his choice to be violent.

ROLE 4:   TO MAINTAIN AN ATMOSPHERE THAT CHALLENGES RATHER THAN COLLUDES

One of the most common problems a facilitator encounters in educational groups is the participants' denial or minimization of the extent and effects of their violence and controlling behavior.

Some men feel ashamed and tell only part of the story, some try to justify their actions, and a few simply don't care that they have been abusive and violent. Whatever the reasons, most abusers deny or minimize their behavior. That is why it is vitally important for the facilitator to confront these statements whenever they occur. The following are common examples of minimization and denial.

- I lost control.
- I just snapped.
- She pushed too far.
- She bruised easily.
- I only threatened her.
- She pushes my buttons.
- What about her violence?
- I didn't really hurt her.
- I got hooked by her.
- I sort of grabbed her.
- Then things got heated.
- We had a little tussle.
- Things got out of control.
- I was only defending myself.
- I suppose she was afraid of me.

- I'm here because the court sent me.
- I never really beat her up or anything.
- I only slapped (grabbed, pushed, etc.) her.

When any participant makes minimizing and denying statements like these, he should be confronted in a respectful manner. In preparing for leading a group, it is helpful for the facilitator to determine how each of the preceding statements minimizes or denies behavior. It is also helpful to make a list of all the ways men in the 13 scenarios do this. This exercise is ideally done with battered women or shelter workers, who are often the most perceptive in recognizing minimizing or denying statements.

Quarterly meetings with facilitators, battered women, and shelter advocates to discuss what's going on in the men's groups in a general sense are a good opportunity for facilitators to ask questions when they sense a participant is minimizing or blaming, but can't quite determine how it is occurring. An example of a participant both minimizing and denying his behavior follows. (He had just transferred to a new group midway through the program.)

FACILITATOR: Joe, why don't you introduce yourself and tell the group why you are in the program?

JOE: I'm Joe. Last July my wife and I got into an argument over money problems. It seems like we're always at each other about bills. Anyway, she was bitching about the fact that we didn't have any money and that we were always broke. She kept arguing and yelling until I couldn't take it anymore, so I told her she had better shut up.

FACILITATOR: Then what happened?

JOE: She kept on yelling, so I grabbed her and told her to shut up or else. The next day I got a court order and the judge says I have to go to counseling and these meetings, so here I am.

FACILITATOR: Do you think you have a problem with violence?

JOE: Sometimes I fly off the handle when she gets me going, but I don't really get violent...I mean I don't think I'm a batterer or anything.

FACILITATOR: Was this the first violent incident?

JOE: I slapped her a couple of times when I had been drinking, but only when I was drinking.

FACILITATOR: Do you think your wife is afraid of you?

JOE: I don't know, maybe.

Even though Joe had gone through the first 12 weeks of the program, he still refused to recognize the severity of his behavior. "So I grabbed her" and "or else" are vague phrases that need to be explored. Getting the men to describe their behavior during a battering episode in as much detail as possible is extremely useful in breaking through minimization and denial.

FACILITATOR • How did you grab her?
             • What else did you do?
             • What words did you use while you held her?

- Did you call her names? What names?
- What did you mean by "or else"?
- What do you mean when you say you don't get really violent? What is the difference between violent and really violent?

Another way of dealing with the participant's minimization and denial is to explore the impact of his violence. For instance, the facilitator may choose to ask the following questions:

- How do you think your slapping her affected how she felt about you?
- How do you think the fact that you slapped her in the past made her respond to your words "or else"?
- Did it make her afraid of you?
- What was the effect on you and on others who witnessed the event?

The important aspect of this dialogue is to get the man to begin to take responsibility for his behavior. As a facilitator feels more comfortable in teaching the curriculum, he or she can encourage greater group participation. The facilitator may attempt to draw other men into the discussion so that they too, and not just the facilitator, are confronting the behavior. For example;

- How do people feel about what Joe has said?
- I'd like some feedback from the group.
- Bill, I remember a couple of weeks ago when you said something similar to what Joe just said.
- How many of you have said things like "I only slapped her" or "I hardly touched her and she calls it battering"?
- You used the term "bitching" when describing your partner's actions. That term is very loaded. . . . I'd like to talk about it.

Another problem is the participant blaming someone else, usually his partner, for his behavior. Blaming takes many forms. A man may tell stories about how awful, irresponsible, crazy, or violent his partner is to rationalize his own battering behavior. His version may or may not be true. However, his partner isn't in the group, nor is the group's purpose to change her behavior. He is in the group to change his behavior. Participants must be repeatedly reminded that regardless of their partners' actions, they have no right to be violent or abusive.

Many men will say, "She provoked me," "She was bitching (or nagging or yapping)," and so forth. It is difficult for the facilitator if the other men in the group defend an action because they too see themselves as victims of their partner's "controlling behavior." An abusive man often finds provocation a justification for his actions and uses his partner's behavior to release himself from responsibility. He may choose to interpret her anger and resistance to his control as provocation.

In Joe's case, he made reference to an argument over money and said, "She was bitching." (His use of the term "bitching" needs to be challenged but not necessarily immediately after he says it.) He then said that she wouldn't "shut up" when he wanted to terminate the argument. To Joe, that is provocation. He can now blame her for his actions because she provoked him. He implies that had she stopped when he told her to, she would not have been hurt.

Although it is important for Joe to describe events that led to his abusive behavior, the discussion should always focus on his actions, his behavior, and his attitudes. The discussion should not concentrate on her behavior. The following shows how to focus a discussion:

FACILITATOR: Joe, you made some statements that I would like to diagram on the board and open up to the group for discussion. (The facilitator paraphrases the situation with the following diagram on the board.)

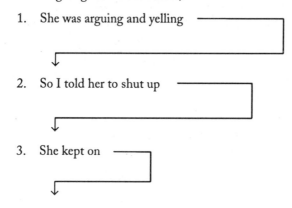

1. She was arguing and yelling

2. So I told her to shut up

3. She kept on

4. So I grabbed her and threatened her.

I'm going to make a few statements that I heard you saying "between the lines." I want you to tell me if they are true for you or not.

- I have the right to make her shut up when she is saying things that I don't want to hear.
- If I tell her to stop doing something and she keeps doing it, I can physically stop her.
- If I tell her to do something once or twice or even more and she doesn't do it, she is pushing me to batter her.
- It is partially her fault that I batter her.
- I had no other choices that were acceptable to me.

As Joe responds to these statements, the facilitator can ask for feedback from the rest of the group. Several of the men (as well as the facilitators) should be able to give examples of how they have used similar statements to minimize their behavior. This exercise teaches another way of perceiving the behavior; explores nonviolent options; confronts the belief system that says the man gets to have his own way (control); and challenges the concept that he "lost control" by demonstrating the intent of his behavior: to "shut her up" when she is saying things he doesn't want to hear.

It is always important to end such a discussion by asking, "How does it benefit us to blame others for our actions?" If a man sees the violence as his partner's fault, then he can continue to believe it is she, not he, who needs to change.

More subtle forms of minimization and denial may also be occurring when, for example, a participant constantly reports that everything is going great in his life and relationship; when he says he is now in a relationship with a "wonderful woman" who is "completely opposite" from the woman he assaulted; when he continually brings up unrelated issues; or when he never talks in the group unless drawn into the discussion by the facilitator.

If the participant is going to change, he must accept responsibility for his violence. If he is not willing to do some self-examination, he is probably not ready to change. One man should not be allowed to hold the whole group back. If a man is continually denying or minimizing his violence, the police report and the order for protection affidavit in his file may provide the evidence necessary to confront him on his denial, minimizing, or blaming. The participants are in the group because they have battered. If a man continues to deny this, the facilitator may refer him back to the men's program coordinator, who will send him back to the court for noncompliance or refer him to a special group designed for resistant and disruptive men.

Another form of potential collusion for facilitators is to let sexist or racist remarks go unchallenged. It is impossible to confront the issues of sexism and racism effectively if the facilitators have not also examined their own attitudes. It is difficult to imagine people not having some stereotypes and racial bias against certain groups of people based on race, color, gender, class, ancestry, age, disability, or sexual preference. We develop these prejudices in a variety of ways and hold on to them for many reasons.

Both racism and sexism are based on the belief that one's own group is superior to another's. This belief provides a rationalization for domination. Racist and sexist comments should never be ignored in a group. When a facilitator confronts such language, it forces men to look at the implications of what they have said.

> TOM: The wife says she's going to—
> FACILITATOR: Excuse me, Tom, but does she have a name?
> TOM: Who?
> FACILITATOR: "The wife."
> TOM: Oh yeah, she does, it's Pat.

FACILITATOR: OK, go on, I just wanted to get her name because it makes her a person to me instead of "the wife."

Tom goes on to finish his story and later the facilitator talks about why it's important to use women's names instead of phrases such as "the old lady" or "the wife."

The following is an example of a facilitator confronting racist language.

BILL: She's going out with this gook.
FACILITATOR: Why do you use the term "gook"?
BILL: It's a term for Vietnamese—you know. I think of them as gooks. You would too if you'd been in Nam.
FACILITATOR: Bill, let's finish what we are talking about, then I want to go back to this discussion about Vietnamese as gooks. OK?
BILL: Yeah, anyway, she's going out with this Vietnamese guy. . . .

After the discussion on why Bill was following his ex-wife, the facilitator returned to the use of the term "gook."

FACILITATOR: I want to talk for a few minutes about words we use for people based on their race, like the word "gook" or the terms used in World War II for Japanese people, and look at why it's important to objectify the enemy in war and how and why we do that in civilian life too.

The group went on to talk about the following:

- How the military teaches soldiers to depersonalize the enemy so they can kill without hesitation.
- How the use of language depersonalizes or objectifies people.
- How language feeds into hatred of people based on race or sex.
- How the men tend to increase the use of degrading language toward their partners before an assault. (If a man sees his partner as "an ugly slut," he is able to hit an object, not a person.)

Finally, facilitators, both men and women, are vulnerable to "getting hooked" by the ways participants minimize their behavior or blame their victims. The following statements by two facilitators caution us about getting drawn into men's denials.

John

One of the men in my first group kept denying any type of physical violence. After five or six weeks of him consistently sticking to his story, I started believing that his conviction was a mistake. I agreed to write a letter to his probation officer to let him end group early. The staff person I asked to type the letter gave me his file to read. After reading the police report and the victim's statement, I was shocked to see that he had not only assaulted his wife, leaving visible injuries, but he threatened the arresting officers and hit his stepdaughter several times. This incident convinced me of the importance of reading the men's files as they join my group.

Linda

I find myself getting drawn into men's stories about their wives if they tell the story in an interesting way. Sometimes the meetings can start dragging or get depressing because of the nature of the discussion. So this one guy, Hal, used to go on and on when he did his log, and I finally realized I was letting him do that because he was funny and interesting. He'd brighten up the meeting, but he was getting away with trivializing his behavior until I finally confronted him on his storytelling methods. Even though I missed his entertaining humor, he got a lot more out of the group once he had to start examining his behavior seriously.

The reality of a men's group is that facilitators could be confronting the participants' statements every few minutes. Some facilitators feel they must do this constantly, and so stifle any chance for critical thinking and honest discussion. Other facilitators tend to shy away from confronting the language to avoid alienating the men or, worse yet, getting them angry. In groups led by cofacilitators, one can continue the discussion while the other takes notes of minimizing, blaming, or other statements to be discussed before the session ends.

ROLE 5: TO PROVIDE NEW INFORMATION AND TEACH NONCONTROLLING RELATIONSHIP SKILLS

Well-established behaviors are difficult for men to change. Even when a group member understands that his belief system is destructive to himself and to others, he cannot simply stop controlling. He must build a whole new pattern of behaviors. The skills taught in the group help the men who have decided to change build this new pattern.

Teaching these skills to a man will be of no benefit to the woman he has abused if he has not first examined his use of violence and made a commitment to give up the power he holds over her. Without the decision to stop abuse and a commitment to forming a new relationship, the skills men learn in counseling or education groups can be used to continue and even strengthen their attempts to establish power over their partners.

When working with abusive men, it is easy to start believing that battering is caused by skill deficiency in the abuser, suggesting that if he could simply learn to cool down, express his feelings, or communicate better, the violence would end. The following story cautions us to avoid this thinking.

Shirley

The first time I met with Jim's counselor, he said, "Jim needs to learn to express his feelings, he needs to learn how to communicate what's going on within himself or he'll keep walking around like a time bomb ready to go off, and you'll keep getting the worst end of it." I sort of nodded my head and mentioned that I had been trying to get him to talk about his feelings for years. The counselor told me that I was doing too much caretaking and that Jim had to start doing that on his own.

Once Jim started counseling, he did come home and talk about how he was learning to express his feelings. The problem was that even though he was talking about how he felt, there was still the pressure on me to do something about it. It seemed that it was almost worse now that he was talking about how he felt. It was as if I owed him more than I did before.

I went back to see his counselor, and I told him that I thought he, the counselor, was doing the same thing I had been doing for years, only he was getting paid for it and that it still wasn't making a difference. I didn't talk about the physical violence, I just used the term "abusive" or made vague references to the fact that I was afraid of Jim. The counselor talked to me about the need for both of us to work on our communication skills and negotiating skills, and for me to work on my anger. Looking back at it now, I can say that Jim always knew the mechanics of good communication because there were three times in our marriage when I left him. Every time I left him, he was perfectly capable of negotiating with me. All of a sudden he could communicate his feelings, he could cry, he could talk about his past, his pain, his anger. He was capable of talking to me about me, about what I wanted, about my desires. Now I understand that he knew what to do, but he did those things only when they were getting him something he wanted, and normally that was for me to come home. I think that Jim never could have kept those behaviors up, even though he knew how to do them, because they weren't sincere. They weren't coming from any kind of real desire to have an equal or close relationship with me.

Several of skills are taught in men's groups throughout the country and have been used successfully since the earliest work with batterers began. Many discussions in group present excellent opportunities to teach these skills. During the first or second week of a theme the facilitator may periodically digress from the agenda to review one of these "techniques for nonviolent living." The third week of each theme of this curriculum is designed to teach specific steps for change. Participants explore alternatives to their own abusive incidents or recreate the vignettes or stories, using noncontrolling behavior. Exercises emphasizing time-outs, self-talk, fair fighting, communication skills, and other nonviolent behaviors are used during the third week of each theme.

ROLE 6: TO FACILITATE AN OPEN AND RESPECTFUL GROUP PROCESS TO ALL MEMBERS

Group Process

Both men and women facilitators will empathize with some of the men in the group. It is important to keep in perspective why the participants are in the group and the seriousness of their violence. The best thing a facilitator can do for them is to help them to become nonviolent.

As the facilitator gets to know the men in the group, it becomes easier to determine which men will respond to a particular issue. Some men are more articulate than others. Some men attempt to dominate the discussion by being constantly intrusive, and others have a difficult time communicating and may resist involvement.

The group runs more smoothly, participants are more open, and discussion is more vibrant if the facilitator follows these group leadership guidelines.

- Listen carefully and attentively to each man's input and respond to both his verbal and nonverbal language.
- Provide positive feedback and be aware of the group's and your own body language.
- When someone is dominating the group, watch for the appropriate time to intervene. Move on without dismissing him or cutting him off.
- Try to ascertain whether someone is honestly exploring his behavior or is just rambling on.
- Give participants positive affirmation for the changes that are occurring in their lives. Everyone likes strokes and acknowledgment for doing something right.

Race, Class, and Cultural Issues in the Group

The more a community is able to reduce class and race bias in the courts and during police intervention in domestic cases, the more diversity there will be in the race, class, and cultural backgrounds of the participants.

The curriculum is structured to assist men in looking at all of the forces that have led them to become abusive to their partners. Although this country is controlled by a dominant culture, we do not all experience the messages and the realities of that culture in the same way. A Native American man, an African-American man, and a white man will bring very different experiences of culture, community, and family life to a batterers' group. So will a bank executive, a laborer for the railroad, and a county social worker. The facilitator must not make the mistake of believing that his or her reality is somehow universal.

No educational program or counseling model is neutral in its orientation. This curriculum is clearly advocating egalitarian relationships between men and women. Its implementation by a culturally diverse group, however, will enhance its effectiveness in facilitating a change process for all men.

Because of racism, creating a group climate that is respectful of all cultures is difficult. There is a large enough Native American community in the Duluth area to offer Indian men the choice of participating in a racially mixed group or in a group exclusively for Native American men. The same curriculum is used, but the facilitators focus much of the discussion about change on examining traditional Indian values of living a balanced and harmonious life.[1]

The institutional and societal support for the thinking that justifies the use of male privilege and control over women so permeates this country that every culture within it has felt its effects. All too frequently programs begin offering services in a community and later realize that the program design is not inclusive of all segments of a community. We strongly urge programs to develop a planning group reflective of the community makeup that can discuss the adaptation of this program and curriculum to the community.

There is considerable evidence to show that the ability to change is linked to a supportive, nonthreatening environment, an environment that is quickly diminished when racism or racial assumptions occur in groups. Programs can reduce the negative impact of race and class biases in men's change process by using a curriculum designed to draw on participant's experiences, their interpretation of those experiences, and their values rather than a counseling or educational model that assumes certain norms in family life and is laden with the values of the dominant culture.

The Relationship of Cofacilitators

DAIP groups are most often cofacilitated by a man and a woman. This has several advantages.

- Two people can alternate responsibilities by having one person do the presenting of materials while the other handles the "process watching."
- Cofacilitating affords the opportunity to examine what occurred during the group. Facilitators can critique one another and provide constructive criticism and positive support.

- Cofacilitating helps prevent burnout. Everyone's energy level fluctuates, and cofacilitators motivate one another.
- Men and women bring differing and equally valuable perspectives to the group.
- A man and woman cofacilitating can provide a model of respectful and equal sharing in a group. It can show the group that disagreements can be handled between men and women without someone losing.

Cofacilitating sometimes requires strategies to counter the perception that only one of the facilitators is "in charge." A male facilitator relates one such strategy he and his female cofacilitator found useful.

Michael

In our group, the men were constantly deferring to me, especially when a hot issue came up or they were trying to get me to side with them because I could more easily identify with the issues. If an issue of group rules or expectations came up, the questions were directed to me. To counter the imbalance, Madeline would do all the check-ins for each group and answer any questions about the program. This small step put her in a leadership position in the participants' eyes and their deference to me stopped. Also, our strategy involved alternating roles. For example, if I was logging an incident on the board, Madeline would be the process person. We alternated these roles weekly, and the group responded to us equally.

CONCLUSION

The intervention process used by the DAIP relies on each person in the system acting as part of a team. The process begins in a private setting on the abuser's turf; continues in a squad car, a jail cell, and a courtroom; and ends in a classroom or counseling center. The abuser is confronted throughout with a consistent and clear message that his use of violence against his partner is wrong and that the community will join with his partner to stop him.

Within that community response the group facilitator becomes the person who interprets all other parts of the system to the abuser. The facilitator establishes the closest relationship to the abuser and consequently is in the best position to help him understand the community's confrontation of his violence. Unfortunately the position of a group leader also affords the greatest opportunity to collude with the abuser. The curriculum is designed to keep the men focused on themselves and the decision they've made to use violence against women. It provides a framework for helping men think reflectively rather than mystically about their past, their values, and their future. It gives each man the tools to change. The facilitator more than anyone else creates the atmosphere in a group that keeps men focused on their abusive behaviors, eliminates the victim blaming that keeps them from changing, and asks men to support each other in becoming nonviolent.

NOTE

1. Information on using this curriculum with Native American men is available through the DAIP's National Training Project. Refer to the note at the end of Chapter 2.

Chapter 5

A Facilitator's Guide to Weekly Sessions

The following themes are discussed during the weekly group sessions for batterers:

Theme One	Nonviolence
Theme Two	Nonthreatening Behavior
Theme Three	Respect
Theme Four	Trust and Support
Theme Five	Honesty and Accountability
Theme Six	Sexual Respect
Theme Seven	Partnership
Theme Eight	Negotiation and Fairness

This chapter presents a detailed description of the agenda for Theme One on nonviolence. Also included are introductions to the eight themes and a review of lecture material for each. Most of the themes follow the same format as Theme One.

Because Theme Five on accountability and honesty and Theme Six on sexual respect deviate somewhat from the basic format, we have included detailed descriptions of their agendas.*

Regardless of which theme the group is examining, the facilitators need to connect the discussion to the men's use of violence and the purpose for its use. The use of violence is

---

*Complete lesson plans for all eight themes are available. Refer to the note at the end of Chapter 3.

not just one of the eight themes. The use of violence must be woven into the fabric of each theme and each discussion. Failure to make the connection between the abusive tactics on the Power and Control Wheel and the use of violence will offer a distorted picture of the role violence has played in the relationships.

In the following story, "Bill and Nancy," the effect of Bill's violence is not dissimilar from many of the experiences we hear from men and women in groups. Bill's use of violence provides a foundation on which he can systematically use behaviors that control almost every segment of Nancy's life. His violence is not cyclical. His abusive behavior is not the result of misdirected or mismanaged anger. When we see Bill from the standpoint of Nancy's everyday life, we begin to comprehend how dominance and survival gets played out every day for the abuser and the women he is battering.

Bill and Nancy

Nancy was 19 years old, 3 months pregnant, and married only 6 months when her husband first hit her. She was stunned. In their 2 years of dating, Bill had talked many times about how his father hit his mother, so she felt especially safe with him. His disgust for that kind of violence was somehow reassuring. He didn't beat her, he slapped her and shoved her down. He left the house crying. She was afraid for him, for her unborn child, and for herself. What was going wrong? Why so soon? This was not supposed to happen.

She went to her mother. She needed to figure this out. Her mother saw the signs of a new marriage under stress, her daughter struggling with the challenge of being a wife, a mate to a man—a boy, really—with the worries of a man not yet secure in who he was in the world. She cautioned her daughter against a rash decision. "It's a hard world out there for a single woman with a child—welfare, the stigma of a divorce, the type of men who would be attracted to you now—your best bet is to work it out, figure out what you can do to restore a sense of balance to your relationship. It's the first big test, be cautious."

Nancy adjusted, she rehashed that single blow until it made sense, until it no longer represented a threat to everything she was building.

Bill adjusted too. He made excuses for his violence. He explained it to her, he talked about why they both had to work it out. He took responsibility, sort of, but mostly he blamed the outside world. He believed himself. It made it easier. He swore he'd never touch Nancy again but he knew she was changed by the episode. She was more compliant—more tuned into his moods, but was also more distant—and something he wanted from her was being withheld. She had taken a part of herself away from him and put it somewhere he couldn't reach.

He obsessed over that.

Their baby was born. She was a mother. He was a father. Another part of her was taken from him and given to their daughter, another part that didn't belong to him.

He obsessed over that.

A phase of their relationship was over, the phase in which she centered her life around him, his phone calls, their dates, his dreams. They lived together now. There was the baby. There were renewed ties with her mother and her sister, who also had a baby. In many ways she was separate from him.

He obsessed over that.

He had become more moody, more demanding. He wasn't violent toward her, but he knew that certain outbursts of anger drew her total attention to him.

Sara was Nancy's best friend. He hated their relationship. One night at a Halloween party, he made a pass at Sara. Suddenly their relationship wasn't so threatening. Now he was in it. In fact, he was in the middle of it. He felt Nancy's jealousy, and he felt the split between Sara and Nancy. He knew he had succeeded. He could stop obsessing about one thing.

On their daughter's first birthday, it happened again. The room was filled with guests, her mother, her sister, her friends, and their kids. He came into the room and told her to fix him a sandwich. He had been working on the car, and he was hungry. She put him off, saying, "I'll fix it later."

He grabbed her by the arm and threw her into the kitchen, "You'll fix it now. I'm hungry now." The party broke up. The tension stayed on. That night when she screamed at him in outrage, he hit her first with an open hand, and then with a fist. He walked out.

She was pregnant again, but she hadn't told anyone. Her world was shrinking. Her friend was gone, her sister and her mother disappointed in her defense of him.

He came home drunk. He decided to tell her the truth about how he was jealous of the baby, her mother, her friend, how he didn't deserve her, how he was scared of being a father like his own. She comforted him. She told him the news, and they held each other and committed themselves once again to love each other above all else.

He became preoccupied about how she would react to his last act of violence. He wanted to know her every thought. Had she talked to her mother? Her sister? Was she attracted to other men? Of course she was. Was she sleeping with someone? He hated the power she had over him. She was making him feel this way on purpose.

He told himself he would never hit her again, but she would have to see how life would be without him. She's stupid, she wouldn't make it without him, she'd never get custody of the kids if she left him. He reminded her of these "truths" daily.

She wanted things to be different. She feared him, she fought with him, she told him what he wanted to hear, she begged him, she screamed at him, she ignored him, she got drunk with him, she started to slip. She started to merge with him. His thoughts and opinions became hers, his truths became hers. She was losing herself, and she knew it. She hated herself.

She had no real friends, and her relationship with her mother and sister were strained. She had tried going back to school, but he put a stop to that. She was trapped.

It was almost 4 years before he beat her again. This time she was afraid as she had never been before. She called the police. She was bleeding from her mouth, and the kids were crying. He was meaner than she'd ever seen him. As the police pulled up to the house, he grabbed her by the hair, pulled her face up to his and whispered, "I know someday I'm going to have to kill you."

The police came. "What happened?" "Why did you hit her?" "What do you want, lady?" "Is this your husband?" "If you want to press charges, call the city attorney." They warned him, "Another trip out to this address tonight will land you in jail, buddy." They left.

The next night he comes home, kicks off his shoes, throws his paper down. He is angry. She doesn't know why, and she really doesn't care. She tells him to leave if he's going to bring all that shit in the house. The kids leave the room. They know when to leave the room now.

They're old enough to figure these things out but not old enough to know why—why the constant fear, the hatred, the names, the attacks.

She backs off when she sees the danger signs. He tells her to make his dinner, and she complies.

He insists that the kids eat dinner with them. They argue. His son argues the loudest. Bill glares. "You smart off once more, and I'll teach you a lesson that'll be hard to forget." Tim tries to appease him, "I just don't feel hungry, Dad." He grabs Tim. "Sit down, now!"

He tells Nancy he wants her to go out with him to a party. She declines the offer.

It isn't an offer.

She doesn't have a babysitter.

"Get one."

She doesn't feel good.

"You never do for me. You must save it for someone else."

She senses what's about to happen. She picks up the phone, he grabs it.

"Forget it. Maybe you would rather go out with your boyfriend."

She tries to change the subject.

He wants to know who "he" is.

"There isn't anyone."

"You're lying. Tell me who he is."

She's fed up. She's sick of the whole thing. She's exhausted, she's scared, she tries to gather her energy to find the right words as she has so many other times. Words that will divert his attention, change his energy. Her mind is racing, but she senses the futility. She keeps talking, talking, talking. Her daughter leaves the table.

Finally he leaves the house.

A reprieve, something worked, she doesn't really know what it was.

Her son grabs his dishes, throws them in the sink, and bolts out the back door.

Jolting her out of a sound sleep, Bill grabs her neck hard. "Tell me who he is."

She can't breath. What's going on? There's that familiar smell. Booze and rage. It's 2 a.m., maybe 3. She struggles to free herself, but she can't move under the weight of his body.

"Tell me who he is."

She's shaking her head. Gasping for air. "There isn't anyone."

The veins in his neck are bulging. His eyes are burning with hatred. "Tell me who he is."

She's grabbing at him, scratching at his face. With one hand he holds her down, with the other he pushes his fingers into her rectum as hard as he can.

She screams in pain and humiliation.

"Whoever he is, he can have you."

She pleads with him to stop.

He pulls himself up and leans over her. "You wanted it to come to this. You always wanted it to come to this."

She's sobbing.

He still doesn't have those parts of her that he always knows she's kept from him, but at this point, neither does she.

In many ways, Bill is very much like most men who are mandated to the DAIP. His acts of violence, if analyzed as separate and unrelated events removed from the context of all his other abusive and controlling behaviors, may appear to be uncontrolled bursts of anger, releasing days or months of built-up tension. He may be seen as impulsive, having poor anger control skills, insecure, codependent, or under stress. Surely there is truth in each of these observations, but from another viewpoint he is very much in control of his anger. After all, he chose when and where and how severely to hurt Nancy. At times it seemed that he felt very secure. For example, when the police arrived, his threat to kill her someday was made by a man who was secure in the power of his violence over her and who felt that ultimately that power would shield him from the controls of would-be interveners. Bill's systematic use of tactics to intimidate, humiliate, and dominate demonstrates the tools of a batterer. These tactics are presented for participants to examine on a personal level throughout the following themes.

THEME ONE: Nonviolence

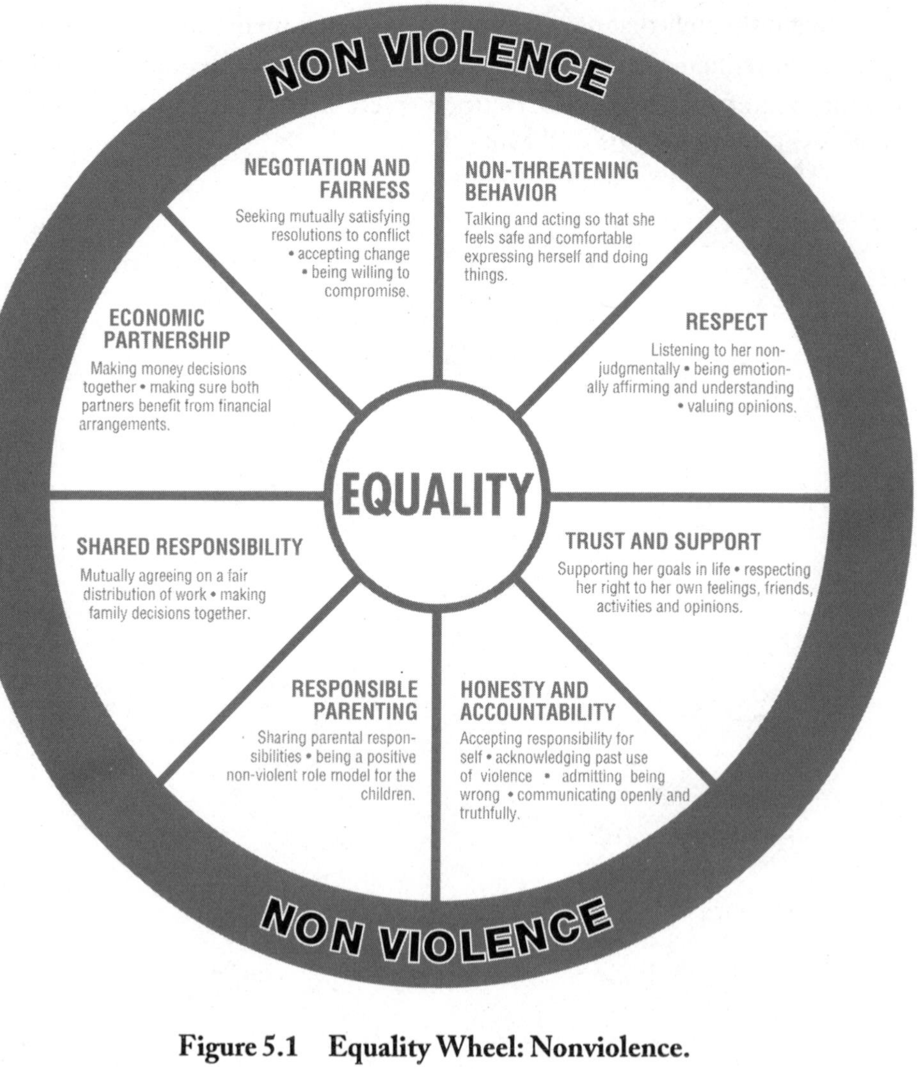

NON VIOLENCE

NEGOTIATION AND FAIRNESS
Seeking mutually satisfying resolutions to conflict • accepting change • being willing to compromise.

NON-THREATENING BEHAVIOR
Talking and acting so that she feels safe and comfortable expressing herself and doing things.

ECONOMIC PARTNERSHIP
Making money decisions together • making sure both partners benefit from financial arrangements.

RESPECT
Listening to her non-judgmentally • being emotionally affirming and understanding • valuing opinions.

EQUALITY

SHARED RESPONSIBILITY
Mutually agreeing on a fair distribution of work • making family decisions together.

TRUST AND SUPPORT
Supporting her goals in life • respecting her right to her own feelings, friends, activities and opinions.

RESPONSIBLE PARENTING
Sharing parental responsibilities • being a positive non-violent role model for the children.

HONESTY AND ACCOUNTABILITY
Accepting responsibility for self • acknowledging past use of violence • admitting being wrong • communicating openly and truthfully.

NON VIOLENCE

Figure 5.1   Equality Wheel: Nonviolence.

One out of four men uses some kind of physical abuse against his partner during the course of a year. Fifty percent of men at some time in their marriage physically abuse their partners. Wife beating and child beating have historically been culturally and legally approved methods for a man to establish and maintain authority in his family. Although the legal right of a man to chastise his wife physically has been removed, cultural approval remains. Use of abusive behavior to maintain a superior status in the family is common in many families.

Perhaps the most difficult aspect of dealing with this issue in a men's group is the ease with which one is drawn into the numerous psychological theories attributing battering to some flaw in the abuser, the victim, the relationship, or all three. An abuser will often admit that he "shouldn't have hit her but . . ." That "but" is reinforced every time it is not challenged.

The abuser bases his actions on two beliefs: first, that he has the right to control his partner's activities, feelings, or thoughts, and, second, that violence is a legitimate method of achieving that control.

Group members often see violence as either a spontaneous reaction to a bad situation in which they temporarily lost control or an understandable reaction to a situation in which they were being wronged.

The following is an exchange with a man who was just starting his group and had been asked to give an example of using physical violence.

ROGER: I only got angry enough to hit her once and that's when she took my car.
FACILITATOR: Are you saying you hit her because you were angry?
ROGER: I lost control.
FACILITATOR: Lost control over what?
ROGER: Over my anger.
FACILITATOR: When you hit her, what did you think that was going to do?
ROGER: Nothing, I didn't think about it—it just happened.
FACILITATOR: We don't do many things without something in mind. I mean, if I stand up right now, it's for a purpose, either to move to another chair or to emphasize my point or for some other purpose. What was it in hitting her?
ROGER: Well, I suppose it was to show her I was angry.
FACILITATOR: OK, if she knows you're angry, then what?
(Pause)
BILL: Would it keep her from doing it again, Roger?
ROGER: Yeah, it did.
FACILITATOR: OK, so you hit her to keep her from taking your car again. Is that what you are saying?
ROGER: Yeah.
FACILITATOR: So, what does your anger have to do with hitting her? I mean, it sounds to me like you didn't lose control over your anger but over her.
ROGER: Same difference.

FACILITATOR: It seems to me there's a big difference.

TOM: I think what he's trying to say is that you're angry because you can't control her. So when you hit her, it wasn't because you were so angry you couldn't control yourself, but because she wouldn't do what you wanted.

FACILITATOR: Thanks, Tom, that's a good way to put it.

ROGER: I suppose it was to get her not to take the car.

FACILITATOR: What do you mean "suppose"? Are you just agreeing with me to get me to move on?

ROGER: No, I mean yes, it was to get her to leave the car.

In this case, the facilitator then talked about all acts of violence in a relationship as an abuse of power, the purpose of which is to control the victim. A facilitator must constantly reiterate the intentional nature of battering, its benefits to the person who is violent, and its long-term destruction to the relationship.

The following is the 3-week agenda for Theme One on nonviolence. For the remaining themes (except Five and Six) only the introductions are presented; their format is the same as that of Theme One.

AGENDA FOR WEEK 1:
DEFINING NONVIOLENCE AND ANALYZING THE USE OF VIOLENCE

15 minutes 1. Check in. Ask group members to report any progress on the steps they have committed to on their action plans. (To review using action plans, see Chapter 3.)

20 minutes 2. Define members' values related to violence using the 10 following questions. (In a large class, it may be preferable to break into small groups for this discussion.)

You may first want to get a sense of what the men's rules are about the use of violence. One method is to write on the board a quote from Gandhi: "Any attempt to impose your will on another is an act of violence." Using this as a reference, ask whether the members agree that using any physical force to impose your will on another is an act of violence. The group may wish to adjust this definition.

a. When is violence justified? When can we impose our will on another?

b. Is anyone here opposed to using force in self-defense?

c. When does that become retaliation or punishment?

d. Does anyone here believe you have the right to retaliate or punish someone physically? When?

e. If a guy walks up to you at a bar and says, "You're the ugliest piece of shit I've ever seen," is it OK to hit him?

         f.   What if he says that and then spits in your face? Is it OK to hit him?

         g.   If someone hurts you emotionally, is it OK to get even by using violence? If our values say no, why do we still do it?

         h.   When did you first observe someone use violence to intimidate and control another person?

         i.   When did you first see someone use violence in retaliation or to punish someone? What was your reaction?

         j.   What experiences have you had that you think influence your thinking about the use of violence?

65 minutes   3.   Explore the obstacles to nonviolence in a relationship.

         a.   Show the vignette *You're Not Going Bowling** or conduct a role play on the following story.

Vignette/Role Play

◆

You're Not Going Bowling

Tuesday night is Jackie's night to go bowling with her friends, and it seems that every Tuesday night Curtis says or does something to ruin her evening. It's Tuesday night, and Jackie is getting ready to go out.

Curtis walks in and starts badgering Jackie about where she is going and how they don't have any money for her to go bowling. Jackie tells him that he gets to go out drinking with his friends and that she can go bowling with her friends. Curtis is aggressive and purposely intimidating. He starts calling her friends she met at the shelter "manhaters" and "lesbians." He pushes her down on the couch, tells her she's not going anywhere, and continues lecturing her. He blames her friends for the fact that he has to go to these stupid groups and for breaking up families and for how much Jackie's changed since she met them.

She gets up to go, easing away from the couch, being careful not to turn her back on him. Curtis gets very angry and tells her she can't go, bullying her, poking her in the chest, and trying to provoke a response. Jackie knows there's going to be trouble and tells him not to touch her. She is afraid because she knows she's going to get hit. Curtis taunts her, saying, "Does it look like I'm touching you, Jackie? Do you want me to touch you?" He backs her against the wall.

Jackie throws one of her shoes at him. Curtis holds her against the wall, and the scene ends as he prepares to hit her with his fist.

---

* The 13 vignettes used throughout this curriculum are available as part of a curriculum and training package from the DAIP's National Training Project. Refer to the note at the end of Chapter 3.

> b. Using the control log, analyze the vignette or role play. (See "Notes on logging" following this lesson plan. To review using the control log, see Chapter 3.)
>
> 10 minutes   4. Lecture and assignment for week 2.
> a. Talk briefly about physical abuse. The following material may be useful.

Additional Lecture Material

What Is Physical Abuse?

Physical abuse is the use of any physical force against your partner intended to make her afraid of you or to hurt her.

PHIL: After I beat her up, we never talked about it except when I promised I wouldn't do it again, so now when I get to that boiling point, she backs down and just walks away.

JERRY: I haven't hit my wife for 5 years but when she does something to make me mad and I stare at her in a certain way, I know she's scared, even after all this time.

EXAMPLES OF PHYSICAL ABUSE

- Pushing, grabbing, shoving
- Restraining her from moving or leaving a room
- Slapping, punching, kicking, biting
- Choking, holding your hand over her mouth
- Threatening to hurt her, raising a fist
- Forcing her to do something against her will
- Throwing things at her
- Pointing or using a gun, knife, or other weapon against her
- Chasing her in a car or trying to run her off the road
- Retaliating by hitting her after she hits you

> b. Hand out control logs for week 2. Before they leave have the men fill out section 1 of the log with an example of a time when they used physical violence against their partner. (The log should be completed before next week's class.)
>
> 10 minutes   5. Summarize main points of the class.
> *Option 1:* Ask each man to identify one insight or useful idea he got from the group.

Option 2: Ask one man to summarize the main points of the class. After he answers, ask if there are any additions.

Notes on Logging
You're Not Going Bowling

ACTIONS

- Drills her on where she's going
- Tells her there's no money for her activities
- Pushes her down on the couch
- Tells her she's not going anywhere
- Puts down her friends
- Puts down lesbians and uses lesbian baiting to make her unsure about herself and friendship with women
- Says she has changed
- Says it's her fault he has to attend these stupid groups
- Pokes her with his finger
- Speaks in a sarcastic, threatening voice
- "I'm not touching you, Jackie, do you want me to touch you?"
- Waves his fist at her, pushes her against the wall, and punches her

INTENTS

- To stop her from going bowling
- To let her know he's in charge
- To make her feel guilty because he must attend groups
- To keep her from having friends and doing things without him
- To make her feel she causes all the problems, she has changed, her friends are trouble
- To intimidate her and scare her

BELIEFS

- He has the right to tell her where she can go.
- He has the right to put down her friends.

- It is her fault he is in groups.
- He has the right to control the family money.
- Lesbians are not "real women."
- She asks to be or deserves to be hit.
- Women who resist male dominance are manhaters.

FEELINGS

- Jealous
- Threatened
- Insecure
- Vengeful
- Loss of control
- Self-pity
- Neglected

EFFECTS ON HIM

- He increases his control.
- He gets to vent his feelings.
- He gets what he wants.
- He loses intimacy and pushes her away.
- She is afraid and resents him.
- She wants to leave him.
- She becomes isolated so he has more power.

EFFECTS ON HER

- She is physically injured.
- She hates him.
- She may be afraid to associate with her friends and to build close relationships with other women.
- She is afraid, angry, helpless, trapped, powerless.
- She is physically injured.
- She wants to get away from him.
- She may withdraw from friends and family.

EFFECTS ON OTHERS

- Her friends are likely to think of her as unreliable and cut off their relationships with her.

MINIMIZATION, DENIAL, AND BLAME

- "Don't give me shit about my drinking." (Minimizing)
- Blames her friends (Blaming)
- "I'm not touching you, Jackie. Am I touching you? Does it look like I'm touching you?" (Denying)
- "You've changed. You went to the shelter, now I have to go these stupid groups." (Blaming, not taking responsibility for his actions)

IMPACT OF PAST VIOLENCE

- She is afraid. She backs away from him at the beginning of the confrontation.
- She tries to reason with him.("You go out drinking with your friends, I can go bowling with my friends.")
- He is able to make her sit down and talk.
- She's afraid to turn her back on him.

NONCONTROLLING BEHAVIORS

- Take a time-out
- Express his feelings to his group
- Take responsibility for his feelings
- Recognize and change his negative self-talk
- Use positive self-talk: "It's OK if she goes out with her friends."
- Stay out of her space when he talks to her
- Speak softly
- Sit down when talking

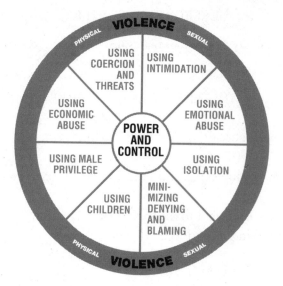

Figure 5.2   Power and Control Wheel: Violence.

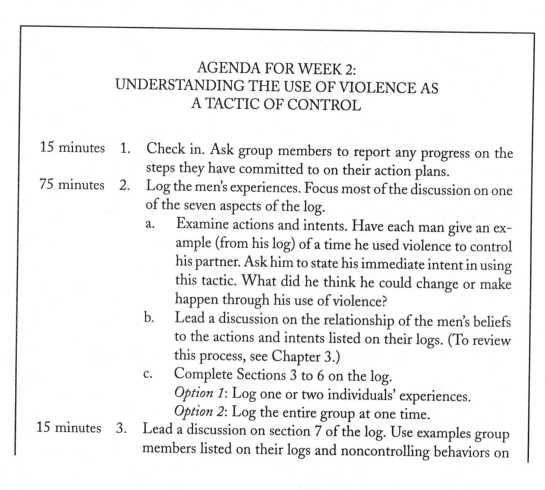

AGENDA FOR WEEK 2:
UNDERSTANDING THE USE OF VIOLENCE AS
A TACTIC OF CONTROL

15 minutes   1.   Check in. Ask group members to report any progress on the steps they have committed to on their action plans.

75 minutes   2.   Log the men's experiences. Focus most of the discussion on one of the seven aspects of the log.

       a.   Examine actions and intents. Have each man give an example (from his log) of a time he used violence to control his partner. Ask him to state his immediate intent in using this tactic. What did he think he could change or make happen through his use of violence?

       b.   Lead a discussion on the relationship of the men's beliefs to the actions and intents listed on their logs. (To review this process, see Chapter 3.)

       c.   Complete Sections 3 to 6 on the log.
Option 1: Log one or two individuals' experiences.
Option 2: Log the entire group at one time.

15 minutes   3.   Lead a discussion on section 7 of the log. Use examples group members listed on their logs and noncontrolling behaviors on

		the Equality Wheel. Covering the rules and responsibilities of time-outs is important.
5 minutes	4.	Collect participants' completed logs. (Logs should be completed before the session.)
10 minutes	5.	Summarize main points of this class.

> *Option 1*: Ask each man to identify one insight or useful idea he got from the group.
>
> *Option 2*: Ask one man to summarize the main points of the class. After he answers, ask if there are any additions.

AGENDA FOR WEEK 3:
ENDING THE USE OF VIOLENCE

15 minutes	1.	Check in. Ask group members to report any progress on the steps they have committed to on their action plans.
5 minutes	2.	Return the logs group members handed in last week. (If someone turned in a log with no thought put into it, this is the time to address the issue.)
45 minutes	3.	a. Ask a volunteer to role play his situation without using controlling or abusive behavior. (Because the facilitators have read the logs, you may encourage a man to volunteer based on what he has written.) Ask the group for feedback. Is the person in the role play still using controlling or abusive behavior?
		b. Ask another volunteer to role play the same situation. Continue to have men volunteer until the group decides that someone has role played the situation without being controlling or abusive.
45 minutes	4.	Use the remaining time to teach specific skills by using the exercises on noncontrolling behaviors in Chapter 3.
10 minutes	5.	Summarize main points of the class.

> *Option 1*: Ask each man to identify one insight or useful idea he got from the group.
>
> *Option 2*: Ask one man to summarize the main points of the class. After he answers, ask if there are any additions.

THEME TWO: Nonthreatening Behavior

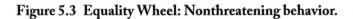

NON VIOLENCE

NEGOTIATION AND FAIRNESS
Seeking mutually satisfying resolutions to conflict • accepting change • being willing to compromise.

NON-THREATENING BEHAVIOR
Talking and acting so that she feels safe and comfortable expressing herself and doing things.

ECONOMIC PARTNERSHIP
Making money decisions together • making sure both partners benefit from financial arrangements.

RESPECT
Listening to her non-judgmentally • being emotionally affirming and understanding • valuing opinions.

EQUALITY

SHARED RESPONSIBILITY
Mutually agreeing on a fair distribution of work • making family decisions together.

TRUST AND SUPPORT
Supporting her goals in life • respecting her right to her own feelings, friends, activities and opinions.

RESPONSIBLE PARENTING
Sharing parental responsibilities • being a positive non-violent role model for the children.

HONESTY AND ACCOUNTABILITY
Accepting responsibility for self • acknowledging past use of violence • admitting being wrong communicating openly and truthfully.

NON VIOLENCE

Figure 5.3 Equality Wheel: Nonthreatening behavior.

Anger is an emotion that we all experience. Men who batter often equate anger with abusive behavior. When men use phrases such as "and then I got really angry," they are often referring to an abusive action they used against their partner, for example, grabbing or assaulting her, restraining her, or shouting obscenities or threats at her. Expressions such as "I blew up," "I lost it," and "I snapped" are good examples of minimizing and denying their behavior and its intent to control or punish the women they are battering. If an abuser can claim that some uncontrollable anger was acting and not him, then he is neither responsible for his action nor able to change.

The facilitator must always challenge the abuser's claim of uncontrolled anger. What does getting angry have to do with slashing tires or punching walls or threatening with clenched fists? They are all actions intended to impart a very specific message: "Don't ever leave me" or "Don't ever talk to that man again" or "Don't even think about going out tonight."

Intimidating behavior intermittently reinforced with an assault makes the violence a part of the woman's daily reality. He gets to decide when punching the wall will change to punching her face.

Once a man has physically assaulted a woman, all his subsequent behavior carries with it that act. He will say, "She knows I'm not going to hit her," when, in fact, she doesn't know that and, in most cases, he himself is not sure if he's going to hit her again or not.

It is difficult for men to admit that their wives or partners don't trust them. It is painful for them to know that their partners are afraid of them, are very angry at them and are skeptical about their willingness or ability to change. In many cases their partners don't care anymore if the men are willing to change because they no longer choose to be with or near someone who has violated them.

When a batterer uses an intimidating gesture, look, behavior, statement, or physical contact, he is evoking the power he has established through past acts of violence.

Sandy

I knew by the way he drove into the garage what he would be like when he got in the house. I could tell by the way he opened the door and took off his boots if he was going to hang up his jacket or throw it. If he threw it somewhere, it meant I was supposed to hang it up and start treading softly. His moods took over the house. The kids had the same sense. We were totally tuned into his moods, and they governed our lives.

Lynn

When he was angry, it wasn't that I thought he was going to hit me, it was more that I knew that everything was going to be wrong. What we ate, when we ate it, what the kids were doing, how loud or soft the TV was on, what channel was on, the way I looked—everything was going to be wrong. I would say and do whatever I thought would avoid a confrontation. He used his anger to make everyone as miserable as he was, and it worked.

Many of the men will be able to identify times that they simply felt rotten and wanted her to feel rotten too, so they picked a fight. What is important is why. They will give a superficial answer, such as "Misery loves company," but it is very important to explore *why*. Why, when you feel down, does she have to feel down too? Why can't she go on feeling good even if you are depressed or angry? One answer frequently surfaces: That would make her a separate person. The following interchange occurred after the group had watched the vignette for this theme, in which Steve stomps out, having been verbally abusive to his wife because they didn't have enough money for him to go fishing.

FACILITATOR: What was Steve's mood before he found out he didn't have enough money?

TOM: Happy.

FACILITATOR: How about 10 minutes later when he stormed out?

TOM: Miserable.

FACILITATOR: Why?

JIM: Because he wanted her to feel bad that he didn't have the money to go fishing.

FACILITATOR: Why?

JIM: (Shrugs.) Misery loves company.

FACILITATOR: But why would a guy want his wife to feel miserable just because he did? Did that make him feel better?

MARK: No, but if she's happy when he's upset then it shows she doesn't care about him.

FACILITATOR: So she has to be miserable when he is to show him she cares?

MARK: Well, sort of.

FACILITATOR: How does that show she cares?

MARK: It shows she loves him.

FACILITATOR: It sounds like you are saying for her to care about him or love him, she has to give up her own feelings and take on his—why?

MARK: To help him.

FACILITATOR: So if she's feeling crabby when he comes home and he just got a raise and he's happy, does she have to get happy?

MARK: Yeah, sort of. She shouldn't bring him down.

FACILITATOR: But if he loves and cares for her, wouldn't he get down and be miserable with her?

MARK: Not if he just got a raise.

FACILITATOR: So the deal is that his moods or feelings are the ones that count. What about hers? Who benefits from the system?

MARK: Probably nobody.

TOM: No, he does.

The facilitator went on to point out how Steve's view of the relationship is based on Cathy giving up her own individuality, even her own feelings.

Vignette/Role Play

◆

You Don't Care About What I Need

Steve is getting ready for a fishing trip he's been planning. He is in a good mood and excited about his trip. He picks up the checkbook and looks inside, and is shocked to discover that there's only $35 in their account. He is enraged and questions Cathy about why there's no money left for his trip.

Cathy tries to explain about the bills and starts to get angry that he is blaming her because there's no money. Steve goes down the register and asks about the checks she's written. He seems OK with some of them and upset about others, like the one she wrote for $35 at Penney's. Cathy responds angrily that the kids needed clothes and that he should pay more attention to what the family needs. This makes Steve even more furious. He slams down the checkbook and accuses Cathy of screwing up his fishing trip, saying that it's her responsibility to make sure that there's money in the account. He tries to make Cathy feel guilty by saying that he's worked hard all week and now because of her, he can't do something fun.

Cathy tells him that the phone company was threatening to cut their service. Steve yells, "Wouldn't that be a shame if poor Cathy couldn't yak on the phone all day!" He kicks the wall close to her (in the video, he tears the phone off the wall) and starts to leave, yelling into her face, "You don't care about what I need!"

Additional Lecture Material

What Is Intimidation?

Intimidation is the use of actions, words, and looks that are meant to frighten, scare, or bully your partner. (Past use of physical violence increases the impact of intimidation on her.)

GEORGE: I guess it was plain and simple, I got what I wanted, whether it was with the kids or the wife. When I came home from work and was in a bad mood, they knew better than to push my buttons.

JOHN: I remember times when I was drunk, and sometimes when I wasn't, I would punch a wall or kick in the door just to let her know not to mess with me.

MARK: When my father came home from work, everything in the house changed. Everyone was afraid of him. He knew what was going on and he seemed to enjoy the power of being in control.

EXAMPLES OF INTIMIDATION

- Giving angry looks and stares that mean, "You're going to be sorry for this"
- Slamming doors, throwing things, punching, or kicking walls or furniture
- Standing in a way that crowds her or standing over her in an intimidating way
- Yelling and screaming
- Walking around like you are about to blow up so everyone has to walk on eggshells around you
- Tearing up or ruining things she gave you or you gave her

The 3-week agenda for this theme is the same as that for Theme One.

THEME THREE: Respect

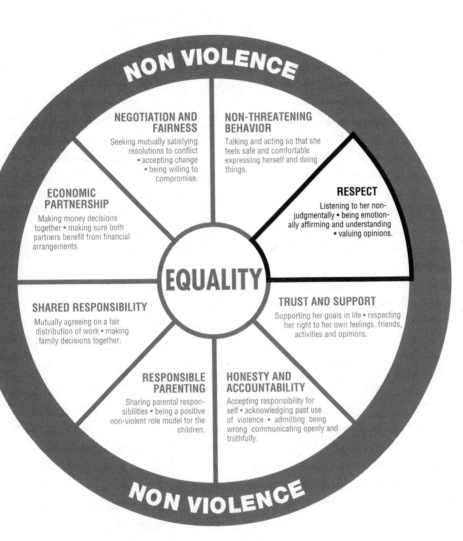

Figure 5.4 Equality Wheel: Respect.

Emotional abuse is one of the most powerful weapons a batterer uses to control his partner. It provides the foundation for the use of almost all other abusive behaviors against her. Through emotional abuse, a man attacks his partner's self-esteem.

These 3 weeks explore two common forms of emotional abuse—humiliation and name calling. They are closely linked.

Humiliation as a Form of Emotional Abuse

John

She was out in the kitchen bitching at me about something, and I told her to shut up. When she came back into the dining room, I pushed her to her knees and told her to bark. She wouldn't do it so I held her there until she barked. I pushed her head up to the dog dish and asked her, "Are you ready to stop acting like a bitch?" She was very ready and she stopped.

(The better the facilitators are at having men describe their behavior, the more likely they are to uncover acts that are painful to hear about. Regular meetings for facilitators provide an appropriate place and time to express the feelings such stories may generate.)

When John reported the preceding incident as a form of emotional abuse, several of the men in the group laughed. They laughed perhaps out of nervousness, but also because of the way John told the story. By his body language, voice and smile at the end, he minimized his behavior. He denied, when asked about his feelings, that he felt powerful when he humiliated his wife, and he said she laughs about this incident now.

The intent of humiliating a woman is to establish power and dominance. It is tied to seeing women as objects and to a belief that a man has the right to punish a woman, often merely for being a woman. In John's case, when he recorded his intent on his control log, he stated, "I wanted her to stop bitching." When the facilitator probed further, John finally acknowledged that by humiliating her, he gained power over her. He intended to make her less than what she was to make her feel powerless. His feelings during the incident were not just guilt or embarrassment, but hate and power. The group spent a considerable amount of time with John examining the intent and effects of his action and then gaining a commitment from him to talk to his partner about what happened in the group and to take responsibility for his action by telling her its intent and acknowledging how humiliating it was for her. The following week John reported on that conversation to the group. He said having gone through all this that he didn't feel any better about the incident and in fact, he felt worse. One of the group members responded by saying, "Maybe that's what will keep it from happening again."

Name Calling as a Form of Emotional Abuse

Abusive men rarely refer to their partners by name—it's "old lady," "woman," "bitch," "the wife" and other terms. This is one way to objectify her—to make her less than human and, therefore, deserving of scorn. If she is not a person, she is easier to control.

Women relate the incredible toll emotional abuse has taken on them as people. They begin to feel deserving of punishment, that they are dirty, nonpersons, or objects.

If a man tells his partner she is a slut, a whore, lazy, fat, ugly, a poor lover, a poor mother, or a lousy friend, then he later can sexually and physically attack her with less resistance and with more "justification."

Emotional abuse is connected to women hating, seeing women as objects, and men's need to reject the value of women and womanliness.

> BILL: This one girl I know—
>
> FACILITATOR: Bill, why do you always refer to adult women as girls? Isn't the person you are talking about in her 40s?
>
> BILL: OK, what do you want me to say, this lady in her 40s?
>
> FACILITATOR: How about referring to her as a woman? This woman I know . . .
>
> BILL: Okay, woman. This WOMAN (enunciated very clearly) I know . . . that just sounds so strong.

For a man to be strong, a woman must be weak. For him to be masculine, she must be feminine. For him to be right, she must be wrong. For him to be in control, she must be controlled. For him to be valued, she must be devalued.

A simple but effective rule some facilitators make in groups is that the men use their partner's or former partner's first name when referring to her. It is surprising how hard that can be for some of the men. It also seems to change the way they talk about their partners. If a man begins a sentence with "My wife says" instead of "Pat says," he depersonalizes her and is more abusive in his tone and his treatment of her in his story.

Vignette/Role Play

◆

Why Do You Have to Come on to Every Guy You Meet?

Jack and Joan have just been to a wedding reception and have stopped at a convenience store on the way home so Joan could pick up a few things. The cashier is a very friendly young man and he strikes up a conversation with her as he rings up her items. Jack is waiting in the car watching them and glaring.

Joan gets back into the car and immediately Jack demands, "Why do you have to come on to every guy you meet?" He accuses her of flirting with the young kid at the store. Joan tries to calm him down. She's been through this before. She tells him that she wasn't flirting and that they've been having a good day, and she doesn't want to spoil it.

Jack won't let it drop. He starts bringing up her friends, especially Barb, who he considers "loose," and accuses Joan of being the same way because Barb is her friend. She argues with him, getting mad and defending herself from his accusations. He gets angrier and screams at her to get out. She leaves, but Jack follows her and starts to taunt her. He yells, "Hey, slut, how about a little quickie?" She tries to ignore him, but he continues by saying, "What's wrong, you whore, you do it with everyone else."

He blocks her way, grabs her by the arm and says he's sorry. He says, "We're even now," as if she was the one who had caused the problem, and tells her to come back with him. She reluctantly agrees. He says he only did it because he loves her, and he's jealous. He says that when he imagines her with someone else it makes him crazy.

Additional Lecture Material

What Is Emotional Abuse?

Emotional abuse is any attempt to make your partner feel bad about herself or any attack on her self-esteem.

DEBBIE: He used to always insist that supper be ready at 5 when he was due to come home from work—although he hardly ever made it home by 5. I always had it ready, and the kids and I would eat at 5. Then I would leave the rest on the stove for him. One night he came home at 9 and wanted his supper and told me to heat it up again. I said, "No. Heat it yourself." He told me again to heat it and threatened me. I heated it. When the gravy was hot, he said he wasn't eating that shit and dumped it on the floor. I cried and screamed at him to stop. He told me to shut up and threw me on the floor in the gravy and then pushed me around in it. I just wanted to die. How could anything this horrible be happening to me?

EXAMPLES OF EMOTIONAL ABUSE

- Calling her names (slut, whore, bitch)
- Telling her she is dumb, ugly, fat, stupid, lazy, a bad mother, a rotten housekeeper
- Making her do something degrading, embarrassing or humiliating
- Making her feel guilty
- Making her do degrading things like begging or eating cigarettes
- Humiliating her or putting her down in front of family, friends, or others
- Throwing or rubbing food or beverages in her hair or face

The 3-week agenda for this theme is the same as that for Theme One.

THEME FOUR: Trust and Support

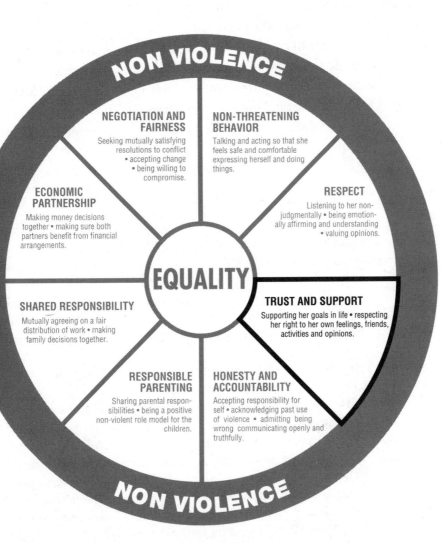

Figure 5.5   Equality Wheel: Trust and support.

Humans are social beings. We have natural desires for companionship, touch, intimacy, camaraderie, community, and friendship. We hobnob, we mix, we mingle, we shake hands, and we embrace, because we are part of a community of human beings.

Many acts of abuse are intended to impose isolation on a woman, cutting her off from a community, from people, ideas, or resources. Isolation increases the abuser's power to define her world, to interpret information, and to force an acceptance of the closed system that he creates. Isolation forces the woman to be dependent on the abuser. Many professionals, family members, and friends attribute this dependence to a defect in the woman that singles her out as a "natural" target of abuse.

It is important that facilitators of men's groups understand how men who batter isolate their partners and the effect of that isolation. Making women dependent is the intended effect of much of the batterer's psychological abuse and physical attacks against his partner. That understanding helps to dispel some of the victim-blaming theories that permeate much of the current literature about battered women.

Gloria

Before we were married, I was involved in a neighborhood block club, played softball, and spent a lot of time with my girlfriends and family. I think Dale was attracted to me because I was so outgoing. After we got married, he didn't want me to go out so much and when I would he would try and make me feel guilty for leaving him alone.

When he started to get abusive, I threatened to leave him, and he stopped hitting me. Our relationship had pretty well hit bottom at that point and I told him that I wanted some of my old life back. He said he would try and not be so possessive and things were actually OK for awhile.

The more I got involved, the more jealous and uptight he would get. He was real upset that I started playing in the softball league again and that our team would go have some beers after the games. He was convinced that I was cheating on him. I had some close male friends, but I wasn't messing around.

His jealousy got real crazy. When I was talking on the phone, he would come in the room or make a face that I was talking too long. During our ball games I would see him drive by the park. When I got home he would start accusing me. The final straw was when we were at the Stagecoach Bar, and he came in and saw me sitting next to this guy. He punched the guy in the face and grabbed me by the hair and dragged me to the car. I was screaming at him and told him I was leaving him. He stopped the car and grabbed my face and put his cigarette out on my chin.

Some women avoid any contact with other men, which means not having friendships with other couples, avoiding parties and bars, giving up dancing and bowling, not going to school, or even not having a job. Many battered women have a very small social circle that consists of family and people of their partners' choice.

Most men in the group will be able to name one or two of her friends he does not like her spending time with. His reasons may be that this particular person is known to be loose, or drinks, or is divorced, or runs around with men, or hates him, or wants her to get a divorce.

The women's shelter is perhaps at the head of the "bad influence" list. The men will often find a common bond when lamenting about the many ways the women's shelter has "influenced" their partners' thinking.

Vignette/Role Play

◆

I'm Just Asking A Couple of Simple Questions

Steve is sitting at the dining room table when Cathy comes home from having lunch with a friend and grocery shopping.

Cathy says hi and starts to put the groceries away. Steve comes into the kitchen and starts asking her lots of questions about what she's done during the day, saying that he called home and her mother's house too, but that there was no answer. His arms are folded, and he is closing off her space. She gives him terse answers and is irritated. Cathy senses that he's not really interested in what she did, but that he's trying to trap her in a lie. He finally asks who she had lunch with, and when she says it was Sara, Steve puts Sara down, saying the only place you'll find her is in a bar or in a bed.

Cathy is frustrated by all of the questions and tells Steve that she's sick of the third degree. He responds innocently, "I'm just asking a couple of simple questions." She become angry, yelling at him that she feels like she's on trial with all of the questions and that she's had to account for her entire day, and she's just sick of it.

She picks up her coat and her purse to leave. Steve grabs them from her and demands to know where she's going. She says, "Out!" Steve angrily observes, "This always happens when you go out with that bitch Sara!"

Steve says that the kids are going to be home any minute, and she hasn't made dinner for them and asks what kind of mother and housekeeper she thinks she is. She says, "You make dinner!" He grabs her purse and takes out the keys, saying, "You're not going, I am."

He storms out of the house, and Cathy follows him screaming, "Don't you come back, you son-of-a-bitch!" Steve comes back to the door and in a disgusted voice says, "I just asked you a few simple questions and now look at you."

Additional Lecture Material

What Are Behaviors That Cause Isolation?

Isolation is not a behavior but the result of many kinds of abusive behaviors. Isolating your partner involves any attempt to control who she sees, what she does, what she wants for herself, what she thinks, or what she feels.

CRAIG: Karen was a social butterfly when I met her, always planning parties, organizing things, picnics, ski trips, class reunions—you know, the one who made that kind of stuff happen. I liked that about her, but once we got married, I wanted her to quit doing that. I don't know why exactly, I just started pressuring her to stop.

      Now I can't even get her out of the house. I got what I wanted but now I don't want it anymore. She's lost her self-confidence. She takes the kids to things but she doesn't do stuff on her own anymore.

EXAMPLES OF BEHAVIORS THAT CAUSE ISOLATION:

- Preventing or discouraging her from having certain friends
- Trying to keep her from going to school or work, or getting involved in outside activities
- Making her tell you where she went, who she saw, what she talked about, what she did all day long
- Listening to her phone conversations and reading her mail
- Not having a telephone
- Making her dependent on you for transportation
- Checking up on her
- Acting jealous or possessive whenever she's around other men, accusing her of flirting or having affairs
- Keeping her from going to women's meetings.

The 3-week agenda for this theme is the same as that for Theme One.

THEME FIVE: Honesty and Accountability

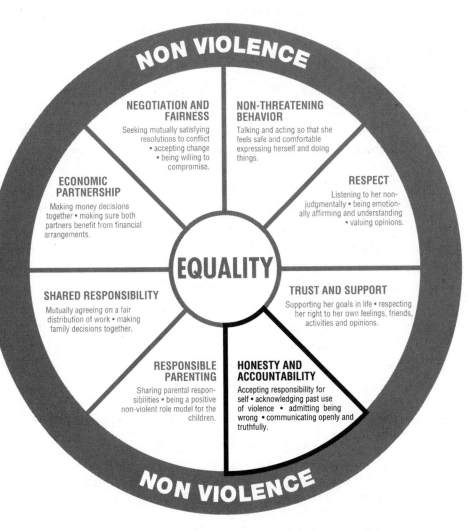

Figure 5.6   Equality Wheel: Honesty and accountability.

In this theme we have drawn on two additional sources to define accountability and its relationship to change: the 12-step Alcoholics Anonymous (AA) program and the Pennsylvania Coalition Against Domestic Violence manual *Safety for Women: Monitoring Batterers' Programs* by Barbara Hart.

Seven of the 12 AA steps deal with issues of accountability. In no way do we wish to suggest that using violence against partners is an addiction or that groups for abusers should use a 12-step model. The AA program is a life path. Bill W. and other alcoholics wishing to stay sober are basically saying life-altering changes must start with acknowledging the past, and being accountable for all past and present behaviors. The 12 steps use the terms "moral inventory" and "making amends." Hart uses the terms "acknowledgment" and "responsibility." Both are defining the basis for accountability.

There are three handouts for use in examining this theme, a sheet on 4 of the 12 steps, and two worksheets on acknowledgment and responsibility adapted from Hart's manual.

Some men will adamantly refuse to accept their need to be accountable. Victim blaming and men claiming to have been victimized by the women they have abused will be common throughout these 3 weeks. The more highly structured these weeks are kept, the less room group members will have to avoid this issue.

No program or group technique will change a man. He must make the very personal and difficult decision to change. It seems so obvious that most men in the groups are deeply unhappy. Change, it would seem, would be a welcome relief from much of the negative feelings, inner turmoil, and isolation most abusers live with daily.

But the kind of personal change this curriculum challenges a man to make involves a long process and a willingness to be painfully honest about a life-style that has hurt so many people around him. No theme will evoke as much resistance or discomfort as the theme of honesty and accountability. If he could bargain with you to see it his way, to "fix" this in her and that in him, he would. He has constructed elaborate walls to avoid an honest self-examination.

AGENDA FOR WEEK 1:
DEFINING HONESTY AND ACCOUNTABILITY AND ANALYZING
MINIMIZING, DENYING, AND BLAMING

15 minutes   1.   Check in. Ask group members to report any progress on the steps they have committed to on their action plans. (To review using action plans, see Chapter 3.)

45 minutes   2.   Define accountability. (In a large class, it may be preferable to break into small groups for this discussion.)

a. Have each man say what accountability means for him or name an aspect of accountable behavior.

b. Distribute the handout (following this agenda) from the AA program, steps 4, 5, 8, and 9.

Discuss whether or not the men think these steps, used by AA members to become accountable, seem reasonable to expect of men who have used violence.

Lead a discussion about what each step means and why it is important for sobriety. Are the same steps important to stop being abusive and violent?

c. Distribute the worksheets (following this agenda) adapted from the Pennsylvania Coalition manual. Discuss whether or not the men think these are reasonable expectations to have of them.

Worksheet 1 requires men to acknowledge fully their use of abusive tactics on the Power and Control Wheel.

Worksheet 2 asks men to take specific steps toward accepting responsibility for their past use of violence. Only a few participants, if any, may be willing to discuss their responses to the worksheet during the session, but it is important to review each point with the whole group. The men will go through the exercise at least mentally. It's also a good handout to give a man at his last group. One way of having him "check out" is to talk again about what it will mean for him to be accountable once he's left the program.

45 minutes   3. Explore the obstacles to being honest in a relationship and accountable for acts of abuse.

a. If you sense a lot of resistance, have the men list all their self-talk during the past 30 minutes. Ask, "Were you resistant to the two handouts and the discussion? What self-talk were you having? ('What about her, what about all my stuff she's ruined?')" Talk about those statements as indications of the resistance to being accountable and the primary obstacle to change. Talk about why it is difficult to admit having been abusive. What does it mean if everything she's reported is true? List the things: I'm a batterer. I'm at fault. I'm the problem, she's not. I have to change. She'll have power over me. How does all this negative stuff affect our willingness to look at our behavior?

If you do not sense resistance you may want to skip this step and move on to b.

          b.   Have each man talk about one person he wouldn't want to find out that he is in the group and why. After the group has generated a list of fears about admitting they have a problem, lead a discussion about how these fears keep us stuck and keep us thinking, "If we don't admit it, people won't know."

5 minutes   4.   Distribute and explain the assignment for week 2 on minimizing, denying, and blaming.

10 minutes   5.   Summarize main points of the class.

        Option 1: Ask each man to identify one insight or helpful idea he got from the group.

        Option 2: Ask one man to summarize the main points of the class. After he answers, ask if there are any additions.

Handout: Four of the Twelve Steps of the AA Program

4. Made a searching and fearless moral inventory of ourselves
5. Admitted to ourselves and to another human being the exact nature of our wrongs
8. Made a list of all persons we had harmed and became willing to make amends to them all
9. Made direct amends to such people wherever possible, except when to do so would injure them or others

Handout: Worksheet 1 on Accountability

To be accountable means to acknowledge and take responsibility for one's actions. The following handout is used for men to acknowledge their abuse and to take responsibility for their use of violence. It is adapted from the manual written by Barbara Hart for the Pennsylvania Coalition Against Domestic Violence *Safety for Women: Monitoring Batterers Programs.*

Acknowledgment of Abuse

- I have physically and emotionally battered my partner.
- I have committed the following acts of violence against her.

_____

_____

_____

- I am responsible for the violence I used. My behavior was not provoked or caused by my partner.
- I have used the following to rationalize my use of violence (e.g., alcohol, stress, anger, other).

1. _____

2. _____

3. _____

- My partner does not owe me forgiveness for admitting my use of violence.
- I recognize that because I have used violence against my partner, she may be distrustful, intimidated, and fearful of me, perhaps forever.

Handout: Worksheet 2 on Taking Responsibility

- If it is her wish, I will limit my contact with my partner. If she wants a separation or wants to terminate the relationship, I will honor her request.
- I will not attempt to gather information about her from anyone or use information I have to harm her.
- I will pay _____ support for her and the children.
  (amount)
- I will reimburse her for all of the financial costs she incurred because of my violence. This includes:
  - Damage to property
  - Medical expenses
  - Moving costs
  - Loss of earnings
- I will not manipulate our children or any other family member to hurt or control her.
- I will correct the false information or impression I have given about my violence and control to the following persons:

_____

_____

_____

Handout: Assignment for Week 2

For change to occur, we have to assume responsibility for our past behavior by acknowledging what we did. This is not easy because we want to hold on to the But: But she . . . But I was . . . But I only . . .

In this exercise list ways that you minimized or denied your use of violence and abuse and how you blamed your partner or former partner for what you did.

Minimizing: _____

Denying: _____

Blaming: _____

List three steps you can take to accept responsibility for your past use of violence. (Use the discussion and the other handouts.)

    1. _____

    2. _____

    3. _____

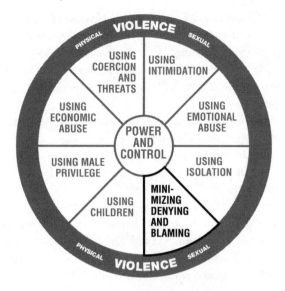

Figure 5.7   Power and Control Wheel: Minimizing, denial, and blame.

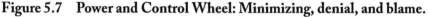

AGENDA FOR WEEK 2:
UNDERSTANDING THE USE OF MINIMIZATION, DENIAL, AND
BLAME AS TACTICS OF CONTROL

15 minutes   1.   Check in. Ask group members to report any progress on the steps they have committed to on their action plans.

65 minutes   2.   Explore the obstacles to accountability and honesty in a relationship.

        a.   Show the vignette *You Promised Me You Were Going to Forget About It* or conduct a role play on the following story.

Vignette/Role Play

◆

You Promised Me You Were Going to Forget About It

Steve and Cathy were at a party last night and Steve got drunk, although he'd promised Cathy that he wouldn't drink again. It's the morning after, and Steve has just come downstairs, hung over.

Steve is trying to be friendly, but Cathy is giving him the silent treatment because she's angry that he broke his promise not to drink. Steve knows why she's acting this way, but he asks, "So how come you're not talking?" Cathy responds that he was drinking last night. Steve immediately gets defensive and starts justifying his actions by saying that everyone was drinking and having a good time, and asks why she's getting all bent out of shape just because he had a few.

When Cathy reminds him that the last time he was drunk he abused her, Steve gets angry and accuses her of refusing to forget about the past. He brings up the fact that she's talked about his violence to her friends and family and asks, "Why can't you just forget about it?" Then he says that he was in control all evening at the party and that the issue isn't his drinking, but her flapping mouth.

Cathy reminds him that her folks are coming to town and that he has promised to do a lot of things around the house. She says her folks haven't visited for a couple of years and that she wants things to look nice for them. She asks him how all these things are going to get done. He becomes enraged, slams his fist down on the table, and glares at her, saying that he will get it done when he's good and ready. Cathy is visibly frightened and stops talking.

---

	b.	Using the control log, analyze the vignette or story. (See "Notes on logging" following this lesson plan. To review using the control log, see Chapter 3.)
30 minutes	3.	Lecture and assignment for week 3.
	a.	Talk briefly about minimization, denial and blame. The following material below maybe useful.

Additional Lecture Material

What Are Minimization, Denial, and Blame?

Minimization:	Discounting the effects of an assault or abusive behavior.
Denial:	Stating or indicating that what happened didn't happen.
Blame:	Shifting responsibility for an abusive behavior onto something or someone else.

DON: I remember the week we talked in group about admitting what we had done to our wives. I had told her several times that I knew I hit her and that I was ashamed of giving her a black eye. The thing was that I only apologized when I was trying to get her to take me back.

I know one guy in the group told everybody in his family what he did. That takes guts. I think he really wanted to do that so he couldn't get away with it again.

You know when you're really coming clean and when you're just bullshitting to go along with the program or to get her to say it's all OK.

FRANK: I used it against her. Every time she brought up something about me abusing her, I'd say, "Look, I apologized, I did everything you wanted me to do, now you're just holding it against me." It took me a long time to get to the point where I could stand to hear her talk about it and not try to shut her up.

KRIS: He never talked about what he did. He kept referring to all those punches and kicks and clumps of hair he pulled out as incidents. Incidents. What the hell is an incident?

EXAMPLES

Minimization

> "I hardly touched her."
> "She bruises easily."
> "I haven't hit her in months, and she still acts like I'm going to hit her."
> "All I did was throw something, not even at her."
> "I wouldn't really hurt her."

Denial

> "I was trying to grab her and she fell."
> "I was acting in self-defense."
> "The courts only listened to her side."

Blame

> "I was drunk."
> "She just wouldn't stop."
> "She knows what will happen when she acts that way."
> "Her mother was always trying to cause trouble between us."
> "The shelter talked her into getting a protection order."

---

          b.   Hand out control logs for week 3 and have the men fill out section 1 of the log with an example of a time they used minimization, denial, or blame to avoid acknowledging their use of violence. (Participants may use an example from last week's assignment.)

          c.   Collect last week's homework assignments.

10 minutes   4.   Summarize main points of the class.

          Option 1: Ask each man to identify one insight or helpful idea he got from the group.

          Option 2: Ask one man to summarize the main points of the class. After he answers, ask if there are any additions.

Notes on Logging
You Promised Me You Were Going to Forget About It

ACTIONS

Minimizing

- Belittles Cathy's anger by making faces
- Minimizes past use of violence: "Obviously you can't forget about it."

Denying

- Controls what issues get brought up, such as his past violence, and his drinking
- Says the real issue is Cathy's bitching
- "I was in control the whole time, there's nothing wrong with me having a drink once in a while."

Blaming

- Turns the argument around, says the real issue is Cathy's bitching
- "The trouble is your flapping mouth and not my drinking."
- "I suppose I can't have a good time."
- "I'm sure your mother knows, your friends know . . ." Steve acts as if it's wrong for her to talk about being battered, as if it's her fault that people know he's been violent

INTENTS

- To make her shut up
- To keep his drinking and violence a "secret"
- To keep her from bringing up the subject again.
- To ensure that he can continue his drinking
- To show her that he's boss and establish his control
- To make her feel guilty
- To get her to lay off him about doing some work

BELIEFS

- He has the right to discuss what he wants to discuss and not discuss what he doesn't want to.

- What he does is none of her business.
- He is not responsible for his behavior.

FEELINGS

- Hostile
- Defensive
- Apprehensive
- Harassed
- Angry
- Guilty

EFFECTS ON HIM

- He won't face up to his violence or drinking.
- He continues to alienate Cathy and her family with his negative behavior.
- She is more fearful of him being abusive.
- He gets what he wants and gains more power.
- He feels reinforced in his claim that he can drink without being violent.

EFFECTS ON HER

- She won't trust him in the future.
- She feels responsible for the problem.
- She feels intimidated, threatened.
- She feels guilty about bringing up his drinking.
- Her plans for a nice day with her family are ruined.
- She is less willing to bring up the issues of drinking and violence.
- She is more isolated from her family.
- She is depressed.
- She feels like a nag.

EFFECTS ON OTHERS

- The children and family feel their tension.
- The children and family are upset by her depression and his angry mood.
- The family doesn't want to visit them.
- Trust is destroyed because he won't acknowledge his drinking or his violence.
- The marriage will likely stay tense or end.

IMPACT OF PAST VIOLENCE

- She stops arguing with him.
- She's afraid now.

NONCONTROLLING BEHAVIORS

- Stay sober
- Acknowledge his behavior
- Schedule the work he needs to do and let her know so she won't worry
- Make an attempt to understand her feelings
- Come to terms with his violence and seek help
- Acknowledge her fear of him when he's drinking

AGENDA FOR WEEK 3:
ENDING THE USE OF MINIMIZATION, DENIAL, AND BLAME

15 minutes   1.   Check in. Ask group members to report any progress on the steps they have committed to on their action plans.

70 minutes   2.   Log the men's experiences.

     a.   Examine actions and intents. Have each participant give an example from his log of a time he used minimization, denial, or blame to control his partner. Ask him to state his immediate intentions in using this tactic. What did he think he could change or make happen by using that tactic?

     b.   Lead a discussion on the relationship of the men's beliefs to the actions and intents listed on their logs. (To review this process, see Chapter 3.)

     c.   Complete sections 3 to 6 on the log.
        Option 1: Log one or two individuals' experiences.
        Option 2: Log the entire group at one time.

25 minutes   3.   a.   Lead a discussion on section 7 of the log. Use examples group members listed on their logs and noncontrolling behaviors on the Equality Wheel.

        b.   Have the men refer to the assignment they completed in week 1 of this theme where they identified three steps toward accepting responsibility for past abusive behavior. Review these steps and discuss progress or difficulty the men have had taking steps to be accountable. Remind participants that being accountable doesn't require forgiveness on her part.

10 minutes   4.   Summarize main points of the class.
     Option 1: Ask each man to identify one insight or useful idea he got from the group.
     Option 2: Ask one man to summarize the main points of the class. After he answers, ask if there are any additions.

THEME SIX: Sexual Respect

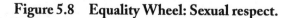

NON VIOLENCE

NEGOTIATION AND FAIRNESS
Seeking mutually satisfying resolutions to conflict • accepting change • being willing to compromise.

NON-THREATENING BEHAVIOR
Talking and acting so that she feels safe and comfortable expressing herself and doing things.

ECONOMIC PARTNERSHIP
Making money decisions together • making sure both partners benefit from financial arrangements.

RESPECT
Listening to her non-judgmentally • being emotionally affirming and understanding • valuing opinions.

SHARED RESPONSIBILITY
Mutually agreeing on a fair distribution of work • making family decisions together.

EQUALITY

TRUST AND SUPPORT
Supporting her goals in life • respecting her right to her own feelings, friends, activities and opinions.

RESPONSIBLE PARENTING
Sharing parental responsibilities • being a positive non-violent role model for the children.

HONESTY AND ACCOUNTABILITY
Accepting responsibility for self • acknowledging past use of violence • admitting being wrong • communicating openly and truthfully.

NON VIOLENCE

Figure 5.8   Equality Wheel: Sexual respect.

Although newspapers carry stories of sexual assault almost daily, marital rape is only beginning to be accorded criminal stature. Marital rape is still perceived within a historical framework that permits a husband to have sexual access to his wife based on the marriage contract "to love, honor, and obey." In one survey (Finkelhor & Yllö, 1985), 1 woman in 10 reported being raped by her partner; in another (Russell, 1982), the figure was 1 in 7. Interviews with battered women conducted by the DAIP revealed that 7 in 10 women were raped or sexually abused by their partners.

Candy was married to Edward for 10 years. Her partner was ordered to the Domestic Abuse Intervention Project.

> I immediately lost contact with my friends when we started dating. I was 18 when we got married.
>
> The sexual abuse began to get bad. He would come in drunk and try to force himself on me in front of the kids. The more I would resist, the more he would do it. He would also come home late at night drunk and want sex. Because he was so drunk, this would last till 5 or 6 in the morning. If I resisted, he would pull my hair.
>
> It got to the point where I would just lay there. But he needed the resistance, so he would change positions or pull my hair. He liked to restrain me by pulling my hair or holding my wrists.
>
> He would bring me into the bedroom and give me spankings or force intercourse. When I would try to get away, he would get physically violent. When I threatened to call the police, he would start crying and say this will never happen again.
>
> He would tell me during intercourse, "You have a big ugly cunt, and your breasts are too small." He wanted anal sex for a while, but then he stopped because he hurt me, and I think he got scared so he stopped. I started to have medical problems—I was bleeding all the time, and he didn't like that.
>
> The more uncomfortable I was the more satisfied he seemed to be. He would set up the situation, and if I wasn't resisting, he would set it up so I would be.
>
> When he put his arms around me, my body would just react, freeze. For a while, I used to think it was just me, that there was something wrong with me—that this was the way sex is. I decided that I hated sex.
>
> I couldn't tolerate the sexual abuse any longer. I was waking up in the middle of the night and would go into the bathroom and cry silently. I got sick to my stomach. I couldn't deal with my kids anymore. I was scared for them.

Men in abuser groups often state that they believe they have a right to sex and see their partners' refusals as unfair and as a control tactic. They interpret unwillingness to have sex as an act of control, and use it to justify their use of abusive tactics to coerce sexual activity.

Coerced sex in abusive relationships seems to be more the rule than the exception. Most men interviewed by the DAIP did not recognize certain actions as sexual abuse.

Examples of sexual abuse reported by women attending support groups in Duluth include the following:

- Making demands for sex
- Making degrading sexual statements
- Forcing sex
- Forcing sex while she is sleeping
- Committing violent sex acts
- Inserting objects into her vagina or anus against her will
- Insisting she view pornography or imitate pornographic acts
- Forcing her to have sex with other men or women
- Assaulting breasts or genitals
- Pressuring or forcing her to wear clothing she doesn't want to wear
- Forcing or coercing her into prostitution
- Pressuring or forcing her to pose for pictures
- Coercing sex in a way she doesn't want
- Accusing her of having affairs, flirting, or coming on to other men, telling her she's dressing a certain way to please or attract other men
- Checking her underwear
- Comparing her body to those of other women he sees or to women in magazines
- Not disclosing a sexually transmitted disease
- Using sex as a reward for being a "good girl" or withholding sex if she doesn't act the way he wants
- Making her beg or feel cheap or dirty if she wants sex
- Blaming her if he doesn't feel satisfied
- Withholding affection if she doesn't want sex when he does
- Expecting sexual access whenever he wants ("It's her duty." "If I don't get it here, I'll get it somewhere else.")
- Disclosing her intimate behavior to others
- Accusing her of being sexually abusive or saying she has a sexual problem if she doesn't respond to demands
- Not caring if she is sexually satisfied
- Telling her that having sex with him will prove that she is faithful

Violence and Sex

Batterers often demand to have sex with their partners after an abusive incident. Women frequently report that they tend to submit out of fear that their partners will be violent again if they refuse, whereas men often believe that sexual intimacy will make amends for their violence.

Some women report that attempts at intimacy after a violent episode made them hope that things would change. The closeness and tenderness was a welcome contrast to the physical and emotional pain experienced after being battered. For some, sex and intimacy after being abused was extremely confusing. "He must really love me." "Maybe the violence will stop now." "Maybe I was to blame for what happened." "He's not mad at me anymore." All of these statements reflect the perplexing dynamics of violence in an abusive relationship.

A women's acquiescence to her abuser's tenderness or sexual advances may seem to him to be her acceptance of some unstated "apology" from him. This self-serving interpretation then gives him permission not to accept responsibility for his actions.

For many women sex after battering is further degradation—the act solidifies his power. Having sex with a man who has just battered feels like rape, an attempt to break her will and spirit.

Emily was married to Dan for 17 years. He was ordered to the Domestic Abuse Intervention Project.

> I approached him sexually, and he wouldn't touch me until I promised to marry him. I believe that was the beginning of the end of the relationship right there—I was engaged to one man and came back down the aisle with another. My feelings no longer mattered. He was the boss, and I had my duties to perform. I had six kids. I saw the kitchen and the bedroom, that's about it.
>
> After just a few weeks of marriage, I said something to him that he didn't like, and he knocked me across the room. That was the only time he was physically abusive, but that was all that was necessary. He was very intimidating. He had an extremely loud voice. It was like I was being slapped with the sound of it. It was hard for me to hear after one of his tirades.
>
> Basically, I was an object he used to satisfy himself. He was the hunter, and I was the prey. He would pursue me and bug me and keep at me for hours and days on end. There was no affection. It was uncomfortable—it wasn't loving or caring or tender, it was awful. I couldn't stand for him to touch me. Just the thought of him made my skin crawl. I wanted to cry when he wanted sex. I felt like a used piece of garbage. I knew that if there were people who actually enjoyed sex, there had to be something more to it than I was getting. There was no foreplay, no cuddling or snuggling. There was nothing. A pretty quick process. That was it. I know he wasn't interested in me or whether there was any satisfaction for me involved in it. He would say, "It's your duty to have sex with me."
>
> When I was pregnant with my second child, I happened to be standing in the bedroom changing clothes. He caught me naked and stood there with this horrible disgusting leer on his face and laughed and said, "My God, you are the ugliest thing I've ever seen in the world." He continued with his laugh and walked out—it haunts me to this day.
>
> I woke up one morning, and he was standing at the foot of the bed with a loaded gun. That was enough for me.

Confronting sexual abuse in men's groups is difficult. During the past few years, counselors and facilitators using this curriculum have tried different methods to discuss this issue, with varied success. We have found that the analysis outlined by Marie Fortune in her book *Sexual Violence: The Unmentionable Sin* provides a useful context for group discussion.

Fortune states that most people have traditionally viewed sexual violence along a continuum. The individual who is the aggressor (active) moves along the continuum and the sexual pursuit remains consensual until the individual crosses the middle line, when the pursuit and actions become coercive. This continuum illustrates the prevailing attitude that it's OK to be actively pursuing as long as you don't cross the middle line when the verbal or nonverbal consent ends (see Figure 5.9).

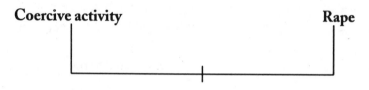

Figure 5.9   Continuum of societal perception: consensual sex and rape.

Fortune further states that sexuality can be perceived along a second continuum (see Figure 5.10) in which someone can be active (and not coercive) in sexual pursuits only if

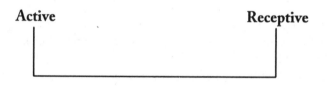

Figure 5.10   Continuum of sexuality: receptivity.

the other individual is receptive. Anything else falls within another continuum (see Figure 5.11) in which the pursuit of someone who is not receptive is coercive. In other words the first continuum obscures the issue and creates a gray area: Is it going too far or not? It should not be a question of going too far, but a question of is it mutual sexuality or sexual abuse?

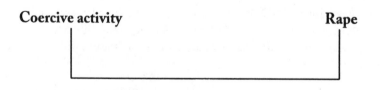

Figure 5.11   Continuum of sexual abuse.

During the 3 weeks of this theme, facilitators use these illustrations to elicit beliefs that men have about sexuality and relationships. In two of the sessions in this theme, facilitators read stories (scenarios 1 and 2) that describe incidents of date rape and marital rape in lieu of video vignettes or role plays. After reading the story, the facilitators ask the men where they think the man crossed the line on the first continuum.

Most men in the group will state that in both cases the man raped the woman, although they may argue about when he actually crossed the line. Many men will silently agree with those who would say that the woman in scenario 1 led him on and that she shares responsibility for what occurred. (The story follows the agenda for week 1.) When the discussion on beliefs begin, the pervasiveness of this thinking becomes apparent. The following is an interchange about sexuality and coercion after the facilitator has read scenario 1 to the group.

FACILITATOR: Jim, when you see a woman in tight clothes, do you think she is saying something?

JIM: Yeah, well, it depends on the woman. I think some women dress a certain way to turn men on.

FACILITATOR: Do you always know if that is what she is intending by her dress?

JIM: Well, not always.

FACILITATOR: What is your response to women you meet who are dressed in a way you perceive to be provocative?

JIM: I'll try and come on to her, see how far I can get. You know, the whole thing is kind of a game. She knows it, and I know it.

FACILITATOR: If she lets you know she isn't interested, then what?

JIM: Well, sometimes I'll keep going, I mean sometimes women say no and they're just playing hard to get, so it depends.

FACILITATOR: Let me ask you, Dick, do you agree with what Jim is saying?

DICK: Basically.

FACILITATOR: How about spending money on a woman as we heard in the scenario—when you take someone out, are there certain expectations that you have?

DICK: Sure, I dated this lady, Kathy, a couple of months ago, and I guess I expected to "get a little" at some point. But I wouldn't physically force her or anything.

FACILITATOR: Do you think that all women realize that this is the arrangement—he buys dinner and she provides sex? What did Kathy think?

DICK: Well, it's not the same with all women. I don't know. How else would it happen? That's dating. That's men and women.

FACILITATOR: Who decides these things? I mean I agree in some respects that this can be a part of dating and when I was dating, there was this sort of game, but I always found it uncomfortable. It didn't seem honest.

JIM: Yeah, but we're supposed to be the aggressor. You know, in the animal world, the male chases the female. No difference.

FACILITATOR: Has anyone in the group had experiences with women where there weren't all these expectations and games being played?

This discussion can last as long as the issues stay focused on participants' beliefs. The scenarios, continuum illustrations, and control log provide an opportunity to engage the men in a dialogue on this issue.

In the second scenario read to the group, the man wants to have sex with his wife when she doesn't want it. He had been violent with her in the past. The discussion reveals beliefs about entitlement to sex in marriage and focuses on the impact of violence on sexuality in the relationship. The following is a discussion after the facilitator has read the scenario to the group.

FACILITATOR: You seem to think that technically Jim raped his wife in this story. Have any of you had situations where your partner hasn't wanted sex and you have?

BRAD: I think that happens in all relationships. There are times when she wants it and I don't feel like it. It goes both ways.

LONNIE: If I was that guy in the story, I'd just tell her I'd get it somewhere else if she didn't want to.

FACILITATOR: Would you see that as being coercive?

LONNIE: No. I've told my wife that before. I mean I don't mind if she doesn't want to have sex once in a while, but if it continued, well . . .

BRAD: I don't know if I would ever say that, but if you're not having sex, something's wrong.

FACILITATOR: What about the fact that in this story the man had been physically abusive? Do you think that had an impact?

DAN: I remember one time after I hit Angie, we had sex that night. I got the feeling she really didn't want to even though she never said anything.

FACILITATOR: Do you think she was afraid to say no?

DAN: Maybe, but I think it was more about not feeling very good about us at that time.

Process of Talking About Sexual Abuse

Although it may at first seem unlikely that the participants will discuss personal examples of sexual abuse, the control log is an effective and by now familiar tool for helping them examine their behavior. If group members are in denial about their sexual abuse, it may be helpful to read the examples provided in the introduction of this theme.

Although the word "rape" is used on the continuum illustrations, the men in the groups will resent any assertion that their coercive behavior could be construed as rape. The important thing to convey is that coercion (rape) is an act of domination and violence. Attempts to justify the behavior in dating situations or in marriage is clearly victim blaming or using sexist cultural practices to rationalize sexual abuse and should be challenged.

People in general have a difficult time discussing sexuality. Sex is still a societal taboo that is joked about or not talked about, partially because of the negative messages we receive.

This theme unfortunately can bring out locker-room behavior in men's groups. Facilitators should set clear limits on how much (if any) joking will be allowed.

- Ask the group if their laughter or jokes are an attempt to minimize the seriousness of the issue.
- Talk about how when we feel uncomfortable talking about certain issues, joking is a way to avoid an honest dialogue.

Groups facilitated by men may have to contend with an attempt to sabotage the group through humor. Female cofacilitators may have difficulty listening to certain attitudes about women, sex, and rape. We suggest that cofacilitators discuss how they are going to handle offensive comments before group and that they process the session afterward.

AGENDA FOR WEEK 1:
DEFINING SEXUAL RESPECT AND ANALYZING SEXUAL ABUSE

(Because the issues of sexuality and sexual abuse are difficult to discuss, the format for this theme differs slightly from the other themes in this manual. In place of the vignettes, written scenarios depicting sexual abuse are read and analyzed.)

15 minutes 1. Check in. Ask group members to report any progress on the steps they have committed to on their action plans. (To review using action plans, see Chapter 3.)

20 minutes 2. Define sexual respect. (In a large class, it may be preferable to break into small groups for discussion.)

Have each man discuss what it means to be sexually respectful with a partner. What are the men's feelings and thoughts about sexual intimacy? Do men and women view sexuality differently? Why?

55 minutes 3. Explore socialization that fosters attitudes and beliefs about sexuality.

a. Draw the first continuum (see Figure 5.9) on the board and state that this is how society has traditionally viewed sexual interaction between men and women. The belief is that at some point the pursuit of sex moves from verbal or nonverbal consent to coercion. Most men in the group will agree with this analysis.

	b.	Read scenario 1 and lead a discussion on the societal beliefs that influence the man in the story. Ask at what point John crosses the line between consensual activity and rape.
	c.	Present the next two continuums (see Figures 5.10 and 5.11) and present the idea that any sexual advance any time one person is not receptive should be considered coercive. Sexual respect dictates that the person to whom sexual advances are made is receptive

       Suggest to the group that if both people are not receptive, the pursuit of sex fits in the continuum illustrated in Figure 5.11. There is no middle line to cross.

| 20 minutes | 4. | Using the beliefs and effects section of the control log, analyze scenario 1. |
| 10 minutes | 5. | Summarize main points of the class. |

      Option 1: Ask each man to identify one insight or helpful idea he got from the group.

      Option 2: Ask one man to summarize the main points of the class. After he answers, ask if there are any additions.

Scenario 1

John and Lisa have been working together at the same firm for several years. Both are single and are friendly with each other and occasionally meet for lunch.

    John asks Lisa out on a date and she accepts. He picks her up and takes her to an expensive restaurant. After dinner and drinks, John pays the check for $100, and they depart to a nightclub for more drinks and dancing.

    John feel sexually stimulated by the way Lisa dances with him and the way she looks in her tight-fitting clothes. He feels he is getting a message from Lisa.

    Lisa is enjoying herself and being with John. She loves dressing up and dancing.

    When the club closes, John and Lisa leave, having both consumed alcohol and feeling a bit tipsy. When they arrive at Lisa's home, she invites him in for a drink. Sitting on the couch, John and Lisa begin kissing, and John moves his hand around her body and touches her breasts. Lisa is receptive to John at this point. John then tries to remove some of her clothing.

    Lisa resists, stating she doesn't want to have sex with him. John feels she is playing "hard to get" and pursues even though Lisa says no and is physically struggling. He has intercourse with her.

Notes on Logging Scenario 1 follow:

BELIEFS

- She leads him on by allowing him to touch her in a sexual way.
- Her clothes are provocative.
- If she leads him on, she deserves it.
- When she says no, she doesn't mean it.
- If he buys her things, she's obligated.
- If she has a "reputation," she should expect advances.

EFFECTS ON HER

- She is hurt emotionally.
- She is hurt physically.
- She feels humiliated, degraded, and used by John.
- She feels guilty.
- She feels violated.
- She feels raped but is uncertain what to do.
- She feels rage.

EFFECTS ON HIM

- He feels sexually satisfied.
- He feels powerful—that he conquered.
- He later feels ashamed and guilty.
- He is afraid of the consequences.
- He may feel remorse.
- He has lost a friendship.

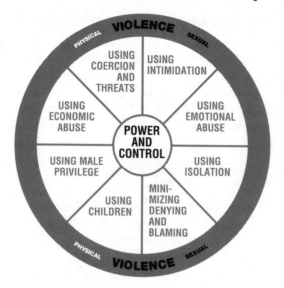

Figure 5.12   Power and Control Wheel: Sexual abuse.

AGENDA FOR WEEK 2:
UNDERSTANDING THE USE OF SEXUAL ABUSE AS
A TACTIC OF CONTROL

Week 2 follows a format similar to that of week 1 using Fortune's continuums. The story (scenario 2) discussed is based on a marital experience.

15 minutes   1.   Check in. Ask group members to report any progress on the steps they have committed to on their action plans.

60 minutes   2.   Explore socialization that fosters attitudes and beliefs about marriage and sexuality. (Because this issue is difficult to discuss, it may be preferable to break into two groups, especially if the class is large.)

           a.   Draw the continuums (as in week 1) on the board and reiterate the concept that society traditionally views sexual interaction between men and women as fitting somewhere along the first continuum. The belief is that at some point the pursuit of sex moves from verbal or nonverbal consent to coercion.

           b.   Read scenario 2 and lead a discussion on the societal beliefs that influence the man in the story. Ask at what point the man crosses the line between consensual activity and rape.

	c. Present the next two continuum illustrations (see Figures 5.10 and 5.11) and put forward the idea that any sexual advance when one person is not receptive should be considered coercive. For the sexual interaction to be noncoercive both people have to be receptive.
30 minutes 3.	Using the beliefs and effects section of the control log, analyze scenario 2.
	b. Using the past violence section of the log, ask questions about how Jim's past use of violence influenced her, him, and the situation. Have the men give personal examples of when they have had sex after an abusive act.
5 minutes 4.	Hand out control logs for week 3. Before they leave, have the men fill out section 1 of the log with an example of a time they were sexually abusive. (The log should be completed before next week's class.) Some men in the group will claim that they have never been sexually abusive to their partner. This may be true. Review the examples given in the introduction of this theme and ask whether they have ever behaved in a similar manner.
10 minutes 5.	Summarize the main points of this group. *Option 1*: Ask each man to identify one insight or useful idea he got from the group. *Option 2*: Ask one man to summarize the main point of the class. After he answers, ask if there are any additions.

Scenario 2

Jim and Jennifer have had an up-and-down relationship for some time. Jim has been physically violent in the past, was arrested, and has been ordered to attend groups. He has not been violent since the arrest. He and Jennifer have decided to stay together, but there has been distance in the relationship. They have not been very sexual.

Jim comes home after work after having a few drinks with friends. Then Jim and Jennifer watch a movie together. When the movie is over, Jennifer goes to bed. Jim joins her shortly after and attempts to arouse her. She tells him that she does not want to be sexual that evening.

He continues touching her and complains about the lack of frequency of sex in their relationship. He says, "You are my wife, and this is unnatural and unfair." He persists and Jennifer stops resisting. Jim has intercourse with her.

Notes on Logging Scenario 2 follow:

BELIEFS

- Marriage means that men have the right to sex with their wives whenever they want.
- Men can't control their sexual desires.
- If she's not being sexual, she's using it as a weapon or being sexual with someone else.
- It's a wife's duty, even if she doesn't feel like it.
- You can't rape your wife.

EFFECTS ON HER

- She feels used and disrespected.
- She feels violated and degraded.
- She feels angry and resentful.
- She feels personally defective.
- She is afraid to resist.
- She is hurt.
- She feels guilty.
- She is confused about her feelings and sex.
- Her lack of trust is confirmed.
- She feels raped but is uncertain what to do.

EFFECTS ON HIM

- He feels sexually satisfied.
- He gets what he wanted.
- He feels initially fulfilled and then unfulfilled.
- He may feel guilty and remorse.

EFFECTS ON THE RELATIONSHIP

- There is more distance between them.
- Ending the relationship seems more likely.
- There is a lack of intimacy.
- Sex becomes unpleasant and unfulfilling for both.
- Trust is gone.
- Respect is gone.

AGENDA FOR WEEK 3:
ENDING THE USE OF SEXUAL ABUSE

15 minutes   1.   Check in. Ask group members to report any progress on the steps they have committed to on their action plans.

75 minutes   2.   Log the men's experiences.

     a.   Examine actions and intents. Have each man give an example (from his log) of a time he was sexually abusive. Ask him to state his immediate intention of the act. Was it just to be sexually satisfied?

     b.   Lead a discussion on the relationship of the men's beliefs to the actions and intents listed on their logs. (To review this process, see Chapter 3.)

     c.   Complete sections 3 to 6 on the log.
        Option 1: Log one or two individuals' experiences.
        Option 2: Log the entire group at one time.

20 minutes   3.   a.   Lead a discussion on section 7 of the log. Use examples group members listed on their logs and noncontrolling behaviors on the Equality Wheel.

10 minutes   4.   Summarize main points of the class.
        Option 1: Ask each man to identify one insight or helpful idea he got from the group.
        Option 2: Ask one man to summarize the main points of the class. After he answers, ask if there are any additions.

THEME SEVEN: Partnership

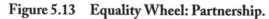

NON VIOLENCE

NEGOTIATION AND FAIRNESS
Seeking mutually satisfying resolutions to conflict • accepting change • being willing to compromise.

NON-THREATENING BEHAVIOR
Talking and acting so that she feels safe and comfortable expressing herself and doing things.

ECONOMIC PARTNERSHIP
Making money decisions together • making sure both partners benefit from financial arrangements.

RESPECT
Listening to her non-judgmentally • being emotionally affirming and understanding • valuing opinions.

EQUALITY

SHARED RESPONSIBILITY
Mutually agreeing on a fair distribution of work • making family decisions together.

TRUST AND SUPPORT
Supporting her goals in life • respecting her right to her own feelings, friends, activities and opinions.

RESPONSIBLE PARENTING
Sharing parental responsibilities • being a positive non-violent role model for the children.

HONESTY AND ACCOUNTABILITY
Accepting responsibility for self • acknowledging past use of violence • admitting being wrong communicating openly and truthfully.

NON VIOLENCE

Figure 5.13   Equality Wheel: Partnership.

Theme Seven focuses on the impact of strict gender roles by examining the use of male privilege, economic abuse and the use of children on intimacy and the balance of power in relationships and families. Ideally, each of these three tactics on the Power and Control Wheel and their corresponding behaviors on the Equality Wheel—shared responsibility, economic partnership and responsible parenting—would constitute a 3-week theme. We recommend that programs able to design programs longer than 24 weeks separate this theme into three.

Many men believe that they are indeed king of the castle; that they should make all the decisions; that they should control their wives and children; and that wives and children exist to make men's lives more comfortable—to be, in essence, personal servants.

When we as a society decide that women have certain subservient roles and men have certain privileged roles, then we also give men the message that they can enforce those roles with whatever tools are at their disposal.

If, as the men in group often say, "Somebody has to be in charge," or "A ship can't have two captains," then the foundation is laid for the rights of enforcement. These 3 weeks assist men in acknowledging the benefits and costs of trying to maintain a position of superiority within their families.

Roger

I'm 45 years old and was arrested last month for assaulting my wife. I had been violent in the past but this time I really beat her up. I don't know what's been happening—everything seems screwed up. I mean, I grew up believing a certain way. You know, that a man's house is his castle. I mean I've worked hard all my life to provide a good home for the wife and kids. I don't think I'm being unfair that I expect the house to be clean or a good meal and some understanding and respect when I get home. Ever since that women's lib stuff started, she's been challenging me—I mean, what am I supposed to do—how can there be two heads of the household? I just don't agree with all of these changes.

While gender roles are changing, many men who batter still hold traditional beliefs that support male privilege. When his authority is challenged, a batterer reacts by employing controlling and abusive behaviors, including violence, to maintain control and retain the privileges to which he believes he is entitled.

The historic oppression and continued subjugation of women in most cultures occurs because men have defined almost every facet of their societies, thereby perpetuating a sexist belief system and institutionalizing male privilege.

Systems built on male privilege provide men with status, power, and the right to make decisions. In the family system, use of male privilege is both controlling and abusive. It ranges from making all major household decisions to demanding the absolute right to sexual access, keeping women in a state of servitude, and applying punitive measures to maintain the status quo. Men's use of male privilege reduces women to objects. The man is the boss, and he will use the church, the Bible, traditions, and anything else to support his claim that he should be "head of the house," the decision maker, the controller of family resources. The effect on a woman is that she is less likely to trust her own abilities and less likely to leave an abusive situation.

Male privilege is not granted by nature, God, or chromosomal differences; it is something that men have built into the structure of society and that they fight to maintain. More than any other tactic of control, the use of male privilege will spark heated debate. Changing societal mores, influence of friends and family, and the women's movement all challenge the "right" to male privilege. The beliefs that surface in this theme alone could take the entire 24 weeks to explore fully.

Intricately tied to the issues of gender roles and male privilege is the belief of most abusers that it's a man's right to be in charge of the finances in the relationship.

Frequently, when a woman talks about what keeps her in a violent relationship, she names fear and economics. Over and over, women in education groups say things such as "I didn't think I could make it on my own," "I was afraid; I didn't have a job; I didn't have an education, I didn't know how to take care of myself and my kids," "I was just incapable of raising my kids alone without support," and "I knew I could go on welfare, but I didn't want to put the kids through that."

The economics of battering extends far deeper than an individual man's effort to keep his partner from working, using his money to control his partner, or arbitrarily making all the economic decisions in the family. Women's economic status in our society is not imposed on them by individual men. However, abusive men often use women's lower economic status as an opportunity to reinforce their positions of power.

Central to any discussion on economic control is the division of labor by gender both in the family and at the workplace. The expectation that women will work for free in the home and for low wages in the work force affects the relative power of a woman in the family unit. Men's work is important, paid at higher wages, and related to production, whereas women's work is seen as less important because it is service related and done for love. Even though both parties are working, only one feels the effect of the status or influence that work brings to him in the family unit.

Often most work a woman does at home is related to the care of children. Batterers are aware of the incredible human connection between a parent and child. Using the children is a powerful tactic when a man is trying to prevent his partner from obtaining a protection order or leaving the relationship. Claiming that he will gain sole custody or threatening to take the children can involve strong protective feelings and may deter a woman from taking action that is in her best interest.

Unfortunately, children often get caught in the middle when violence and abuse occurred in a relationship. They are frequently confused, torn, and traumatized as they are forced to choose one parent or the other.

Many men who batter are loving and caring fathers, and would not consciously use their children as weapons against their partners or former partners. However, some men who batter recognize that the children are the last part of her life that he can still control.

The issues that surface in discussions during this theme are not only about behaviors and men's choices to use certain tactics to "get their way." These issues are about who men are in relationship to women. If discussed in depth, the material in these 3 weeks can shake the foundation of a man's perceived right to impose his will on the woman he batters.

To accommodate the issues of partnership discussed in the theme, we suggest that you role play all three scenarios or show all three video vignettes. As you log the scenes in week 1, log three sets of actions: using male privilege, using economic abuse, and using children. Then as you move on through the log, combine the three discussions. What are some intents of all three men in the scenarios? What were some beliefs of all three men? Ask the men to pick one of the three topics to complete their logs for week 2.

Vignette/Role Play (Using Male Privilege)

◆

Eat at Kimo's

Curtis comes home late after he's been drinking with his friend Kimo. He starts arguing with his wife Jackie about how he felt that she put him down because he doesn't have a job. Jackie denies that was her intent and that she was just telling their friends what her life was like.

Jackie states that she is tired and wants to go to bed, but Curtis insists on talking. He tells Jackie, "You always want to talk, well tonight we're going to talk." Jackie doesn't challenge Curtis because he is intoxicated and belligerent. The discussion degenerates, and Jackie repeats that she's tired and wants to go to bed. At this point, Curtis demands dinner. Jackie is upset at the late-night request and reminds him that dinner was ready hours ago. Curtis replies, "What is it, Jackie, are you too good to make your husband dinner?"

Vignette/Role Play (Using Male Privilege and Economic Abuse)

◆

Going to School Doesn't Make You Smart

Cathy has decided to go back to college, and she's excited about it. She knows this decision is going to upset Steve, and for a long time has avoided the issue. But now that he's going to his men's group, she thinks this is a good time to deal with it. Steve is coming home from work, and Cathy is sitting on the couch with the college catalog next to her.

Steve comes in, sits next to Cathy, and takes his shoes off. Then he notices the catalog, and his mood immediately changes. He asks, "What's this?" Cathy tells him it's the college catalog and that she's ready to go back to school. He accuses her of checking this stuff out without talking to him first, as if she's been sneaking around behind his back. He starts to quiz her. "How are you going to get there? Who's going to take the kids to day care? How are we going to pay for you to go back? Who's going to clean house?"

Cathy answers all of his questions, hoping that she can convince him that this is not only good for her, but that it will also be good for them. Steve tells her not to expect him to help out on this, and he's not changing a thing in his life, but that if she wants to get her "little degree," to go ahead. Then he says, "Going to school is really dumb—you'd just be wasting time there." Cathy tries to answer him but he becomes sarcastic and says that going to school doesn't make you smart or even qualify you for a job. She asks him why he is so threatened by the idea. He throws the catalog back onto the couch and denies that he's threatened. Then he asks her, "What are you going to be, a bank president or an accountant? You can't even keep our checkbook straight!"

Cathy feels angry and disappointed and becomes withdrawn. She realizes how difficult he is going to make things, and she tells him, "OK, Steve, I won't go." He says, "Look, I didn't say you couldn't go, did I?"

Vignette/Role Play (Using Children)

◆

You'd Better Start Thinking About What You're Doing to Our Son

Larry is getting ready to leave for work. Jan tells him not to come back tonight because he was violent again. He tries to minimize what happened, but Jan reminds him that her arms are black and blue from the last assault and is insistent that Larry not return.

Larry becomes defensive and tells Jan that her reaction (kicking him out) will have a negative impact on their son. He tries to make her feel guilty by implying that Jan is depriving their son of a father. His closing statement is, "You'd better start thinking about what you're doing to our son."

Additional Lecture Material

What Is Male Privilege?

Male privilege is a belief system that contends that you as a man are entitled to certain privileges simply because you are male.

NORMA: When he would come home the whole feel of the house would change. The TV would be turned to his channel. If he didn't want the kids around he would tell me to get rid of them, and I always had to ask him when he wanted dinner. Because I didn't want to upset him I played the game.

TOM: There are certain jobs that are woman's work. I can't cook, I hate housework, and a lot of the stuff with the kids she is better at. There are things that I do better because I learned as a kid, like working on cars. Men's and women's roles have been the same since the beginning of time, and I don't see any reason to change now.

FRAN: He always throws the Bible stuff up in my face. He just tells me that it's my duty to obey.

EXAMPLES OF MALE PRIVILEGE

- Insisting on making the major decisions
- Having the final say on how the money gets spent
- Having the right to define family roles
- Expecting women to accept male authority in relationships
- Being able to set and change the rules
- Treating your partner like a servant
- Expecting to have sex when you want it

What Is Using the Children?

Using the children is any attempt to control your partner by threatening or damaging her relationship with her children.

TYRONE: I used to tell Susan that if she left me she would never see the kids again. I told her that I would move to another state, and I would change our names. I wouldn't have done it, but I really think she was convinced that I would.

DENISE: I don't know what to do now. I thought the worst of it was over since he's been excluded from the house. But I still have to have ongoing contact with him over visitation. I'm scared every time I have to drop the kids off or when he returns them wondering what he might do.

LONNIE: Every time I had the kids for visitation, I would try and trick them into telling me about their mother, especially what men she was seeing. I would then confront her with this information and threaten to use it in court.

EXAMPLES OF USING THE CHILDREN

- Making her feel guilty about the children
- Telling her that she is an unfit mother
- Threatening to call child protection
- Using the children to relay messages
- Using visitation to harass her
- Threatening to take the children and never let her see them
- Telling the children lies or negative things about their mother
- Interrogating the children about what their mother does or who she sees

What Is Economic Abuse?

Economic abuse is using control of the family income or limiting your partner's access to money to keep her dependent on you or to get your own way.

CANDI: At first he didn't care about my part-time job, but when I got a promotion everything seemed to change. I don't know if he was threatened, but he hated the fact that I was working and making more money, even though it benefited both of us.

JERRY: I warned her that if we didn't get out of debt there were going to be consequences. It was like she didn't care because she would make long-distance phone calls to her family. I finally closed all our charge accounts, cut up the credit cards, and had the phone removed. She shouldn't complain because I warned her that something had to be done about this debt.

AMY: I felt like a kid having to ask for money from him. When I would buy anything I had to justify the expense and he rarely approved. Even though I was financially contributing, it was like it was his money.

EXAMPLES OF ECONOMIC ABUSE

- Preventing her from getting a job
- Sabotaging her existing job through harassment
- Making her quit a job
- Making her ask for money
- Making her give him her paycheck
- Giving her an allowance
- Taking her credit cards
- Not letting her know about or have access to family income
- Accusing her of hiding money

The 3-week agenda for this theme is the same as that for Theme One.

THEME EIGHT: Negotiation and Fairness

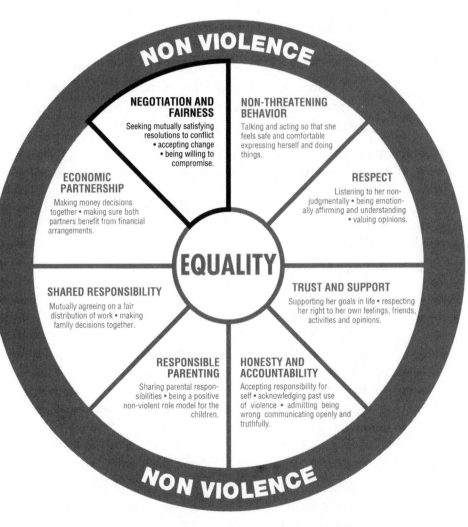

Figure 5.14   Equality Wheel: Negotiation and fairness.

In almost all groups for men who batter, the facilitators teach some kind of negotiating skills. Although it is obvious that many men who batter do not have much experience in negotiating, preconditions to teaching these skills are often ignored in working with abusive men. The goal of negotiation is to balance the needs of two parties and to reach a resolution that is mutually satisfactory.

Teaching men the language and rules of fair negotiating can backfire unless participants first acknowledge that most decisions they want to negotiate are not their decisions to negotiate.

The following is an exchange following a role play of *Going to School Doesn't Make You Smart*, in which Steve is attempting to keep Cathy from going to school. Steve does this by throwing up all sorts of obstacles ("What about the kids?" "How are you going to get there?" "How will we pay for it?" "What good will it do for you to go to school?"). Cathy has resolved all of these problems, so Steve then shifts tactics and attacks her self-image. One man has just finished role playing with the facilitator and the group is giving feedback. Most of the men found him to be just as controlling as Steve was in the video.

> LOUIS: Well, he didn't try to compromise with her at all. It was just all his way.
> FACILITATOR: OK, Louis, why don't you and Warren trade places, and we'll do it again.

Louis sits down next to the facilitator and ask a few questions about the college catalog. She says she's going to sign up for a few classes in the fall to finish getting her accounting degree and to do something intellectually stimulating.

> LOUIS: Have you considered a correspondence course?
> FACILITATOR: What?
> LOUIS: A correspondence course.
> FACILITATOR: Why would I want to take a correspondence course? I want to be with people, Louis. I need to get back into circulation. I've been at home with three kids for 6 years.
> LOUIS: A correspondence course would let you finish your degree, and the children wouldn't be without their mother. You can get into circulation when you get a job.
> FACILITATOR: Louis, part of the reason I want to go to school is to be with people, to start thinking and using my mind. How can I do that on the pen-pal plan?
> LOUIS: Couldn't you get some lady friends who are interested in accounting to meet here once a week to study together? That would get you with people and keep you with the kids. I could watch them on your study night.

At this point the facilitator stopped the role play and asked for feedback: "Was Louis negotiating fairly?" The overwhelming response was yes, that he was trying to compromise, but she was only going to have it her way. Thirty minutes earlier, this group had viewed *Going to School Doesn't Make You Smart* and concluded that the only reason Steve didn't want Cathy to go to school was because Cathy would meet other men there and would have improved self-esteem if she was getting good grades and positive feedback from others.

The question for the group then becomes not how can the man negotiate, but what is negotiable?

- Whether or not she goes back to school?
- How she goes (i.e., correspondence or attendance)?
- Who will care for the children when she's gone?
- How will the schooling be paid for?
- Who will have use of the car on her school days?

Most of the issues men will want to negotiate with their partners will not be negotiable. For example, for most women, the following points are solely their decisions and therefore not negotiable:

- Whether or not she continues her protection order
- Whether or not she enters another relationship
- Whether or not she works outside the home
- Whether or not she spends time with those of her friends he doesn't like
- Whether or not she attends women's support groups

Much of what the men will want to see as compromise is really another way of controlling their partners. The facilitator must constantly bring this out in the groups.

Threats and Coercion

Every day we read in the newspaper or hear on the news about men who carry out their threats—husbands who have shot and killed their wives and children after a divorce or separation. Abusers frequently destroy property or even kill pets as a warning about what will happen to her if she leaves him.

Threats, like intimidation, are used to immobilize the woman. She can't leave because she believes he'll find her and hurt her. If she gets help from others, they will be in danger too. So she stays and he gains more power over her.

About half the women in education groups tell about men making suicide threats, yet when men are asked about these threats they play down their impact, deny making them, or say they weren't serious.

Threats and coercion terrorize women and become very effective tactics of control.

It is extremely difficult for most men to admit to threatening and coercing their partners. With few exceptions, women who live with abusive partners report a whole continuum of coercive behaviors. On one end of that continuum, men are coercing women to do things for them, to go places they don't want to go, to invite people over they don't want to see, to leave places when they are enjoying themselves. At the other end of the

continuum, women are coerced into doing things totally against their will such as prostitution, using drugs, shoplifting, or writing bad checks.

Men's use of threats and coercion is often described by women as the most devastating
of battering incidents.

Threats are used to place the woman in fear of something horrible happening if she
doesn't do what he wants. The threat allows the coercion to be effective. The fear doesn't
go away like a black eye or the pain from a bruised rib. The fear from these threats stays
with her day in and day out.

Nancy

One night Mark sat at the kitchen table for over two hours with a gun to his head. First he
would talk very quietly and calmly and then he'd start yelling and the next minute he'd be
sobbing. I said whatever I thought would keep him from pulling the trigger. Finally, he got
up and said goodbye and walked out the door. About a minute later I heard the shot. I
grabbed the kids and put them all up in the bedroom and told them to just wait for me. They
were crying and Lisa was shaking so badly, she bit her lip, and it was bleeding. I ran out the
back door, and Mark was sitting on the hood of his car. He grinned at me and said, "I just
wanted to see if you cared enough to come out and look."

It is difficult to imagine the night of terror this woman and her children lived through.
It is equally difficult to imagine the effects of the rage she must feel and how unsafe it is
for her to express it. More than half of the women in the women's educational groups
report that their partners have threatened suicide.

Another common threat, often even more powerful, is a man's threat to gain custody
of the children or kidnap them if his partner leaves him. Women are particularly vulnerable to threats regarding their children. If a woman has been battered during a long period, her partner may be able to strengthen the threat of getting custody by referring to the
fact that she has seen a psychiatrist or therapist or has abused alcohol. She may have left
the home in fear after being abused and not taken her children. He tells her that is aban-
donment and claims the court will award him custody. Whether or not his claims that he
will have a better chance of getting custody are valid, they are powerful weapons to force
a woman's submission.

Threats are more difficult for many women to cope with than physical attacks because
they are less visible. When a man chokes a woman, her body responds instantly: It tight-
ens, her heart beats faster, she grabs his hands, she cringes in pain and fear. He says what
he has to say, makes his demands, and then lets go. Her body slumps, she cries, her fear
lessens. His threat of taking the children stays with her in a different way. It's as if he has
grabbed her throat with invisible hands, and he isn't letting go. Days go by, and her fear

throbs in some corner of her mind and spirit. She walks through the day, the week, the month being choked by hands nobody sees, nobody acknowledges.

It is important for facilitators to listen to the stories of women who are threatened to understand the full impact of men's use of threats.

Terrifying Acts

The abuser escalates his abuse by committing terrifying acts to carry out his threats.

Michelle

Tim came in the house one day with this weird look on his face. He knew I had been thinking of a divorce. He told me to go out and clean the garage. I knew something was wrong so I didn't challenge him or argue with him. I went out to the garage, and our dog was laying dead. Tim beat him to death with a two-by-four. He had told me for months that he would kill the dog if I didn't keep him from shedding on the carpeting. I think things were never the same after that. Tim was letting me know that if I left him he'd kill me. I didn't leave him for 4 more years, and a month after I did leave, he tried to kill me. It's been 4 years since he got out of jail, and I still believe he may kill me someday.

For many women, the threat of losing their children becomes a reality. Children are taken for days, months, or years, and in some cases their mother never sees them again. Pets are killed, friends and family are harassed and injured, fires set, cars or houses destroyed, and suicides and homicides are carried out.

Vignette/Role Play

◆

No Judge Is Going to Give You Custody of Our Kids

Cathy has taken out a civil protection order against Steve because of his abuse. The hearing is scheduled for the next day. She is cleaning the house and is bringing the garbage out back, where she finds Steve. He's been waiting for her.

Cathy sees Steve and panics. She tells him to leave or she'll call the police, that the protection order says he isn't supposed to be on the property. Steve stands outside the fence and pleads with her to talk. He seems calm, so Cathy stays and starts to talk with him. Steve assures her that she doesn't have to be afraid and that he wants to work things out. "I really love you, Cath—I'm sorry about the stuff I've done. You mean everything to me, babe—I couldn't live without you."

Cathy says that things would have to change and that Steve would have to get some help. She tells him, "Maybe we can work things out, but right now, I just need some time." When Steve hears this, he realizes that she's not going to drop the protection order and he becomes enraged, yelling, "I can't believe you have a court order against your own husband!" His whole body is tense and intimidating. He is furious and tells her that she's wrecking their marriage by taking out the order, and that they are finished if she goes ahead with it.

Cathy realizes that there's no point in talking any more and starts to walk back to the house. Steve starts screaming insults and threats. "I'll get custody of the kids, you can be damn sure! You've gone to a shrink! No judge is going to give you custody of the kids! No way, not the kind of wife and mother you are!" Cathy covers her ears and keeps walking. He keeps yelling at her, asking how she would support herself and saying that she doesn't know how to do anything. "Our marriage is over—you're the only one who can stop this!"

Additional Lecture Material

What Are Coercion and Threats?

Making threats or using coercion is saying or doing something to make your partner afraid that something bad will happen to her if she doesn't do what you want. It's like blackmail.

EXAMPLES OF COERCION AND THREATS

- "If you leave me, I'll kill any man who even looks at you."
- "If you leave, I'll get custody of the kids."
- "If you don't drop that order for protection, I'll call welfare and report you for fraud."
- "If you call the cops, I'll divorce you, and you'll never see me or your kids again."
- "I'll never pay you 1 cent of child support."
- "If you leave me, I'll kill myself."
- Driving recklessly with her in the car until she says or does what you want
- Forcing her to write bad checks, steal, use drugs or alcohol, have sex with someone else

Mark

I used to threaten Barbara a lot about the kids. She was afraid of losing them because she had a baby in high school and was forced to give it up for adoption. I never really wanted total custody of the kids but when she filed for divorce, I told my lawyer to go for full custody.

Looking back, I can see now that all the time I spent in court accusing her of being a bad mother was just to punish her for leaving me. It didn't help get her back or help in my relationship with the kids. Two of the kids wouldn't even talk to me after the divorce.

One night, just to punish Barb, I told the kids their mom had an illegitimate child. It hurt everyone. I guess the kids suffered a lot. I finally had to tell them that I was using all that custody stuff and telling them about the adoption because I wanted to hurt their mother. It's better now with the kids, but it will be a long time for things to be right again.

Vicki

He got into all these drug deals. He was in way over his head, so he needed money. He made me write bad checks, steal, and, finally, he became my pimp.

The facilitator may also decide to use the following negotiation exercises during week 3 of this theme.

The 3-week agenda for this theme is the same as that for Theme One.

Handout: What Is Open to Negotiation?

An issue is open to negotiation if it is not entirely one person's right to decide. It's open to discussion, but not negotiation, if it is only one person's right to decide.

If you think an item in Table 5.1 should be open to negotiation, check box 1. If you think it is open for discussion and input but not negotiation, because your partner has the right to make the decision, check box 2. If you think it is open for discussion and input but not negotiation, because it is your right to make the decision, check box 3.

TABLE 5.1
What Is Open to Negotiation?

	Open—both decide	Not open—partner decides	Not open—you decide
1. Which friends can she spend time with? Which friends can you spend time with?			
2. Who cooks/cleans on weekdays?			
3. Who cooks/cleans on weekends?			
4. Will she drink/use drugs again? Will you drink/use drugs again?			
5. Will she drink on certain occasions? Will you drink on certain occasions?			
6. Who finds a sitter for the children?			
7. Will you buy a car/truck with your own money?			
8. Will she buy a car/truck with her own money?			
9. Will she get a job or change jobs? Will you get a job or change jobs?			
10. Will she go to school? Will you go to school?			
11. Which friends or relatives can visit your home?			
12. How will the children be disciplined?			
13. When will the children be disciplined?			
14. Can she go on a trip without you? Can you go on a trip without her?			
15. What is your paycheck spent on? What is her paycheck spent on?			

Handout: Negotiation Skills

1. *Being prepared*:   Before people can even begin the process of negotiation, they must first be committed to a fair process. In preparation for being fair the parties must be ready to

- listen
- reach a mutually satisfying resolution
- hear things they disagree with or find painful without reacting abusively or defensively
- accept that something will change

2. *Setting some rules*:   Begin by reviewing these rules and adding any that you mutually decide are important.

- No yelling
- No bringing up unrelated issues
- No using threats or intimidation
- No playing mind games
- Is a time limit needed for this discussion?
- Is a third party needed to help with this discussion?

3. *Defining the problem:*   What are we negotiating? Is this negotiable?

- How does each person experience and define the problem? (This will be different for each person.)
- Who else is affected and how?

4. *Identifying goals*:   Short- and long-term goals should be identified.

- *Short-term*: Name the things that need to be included in an immediate solution.
- *Long-term*: Name the things that need to be included in a final solution.

5. *Finding solutions*:   What would each person propose as an immediate and a long-term solution that addresses the things each person has said need to be considered:

- Is compromise necessary or can both parties be satisfied?
- If compromise is necessary, list several fair solutions.

REFERENCES

Finkelhor, D., & Yllö, K. (1985). *License to Rape: Sexual Abuse of Wives.* New York: Holt, Rinehart, & Winston.
Fortune, M. (1983). *Sexual Violence: The Unmentionable Sin.* New York: Pilgrim Press.
Russell, D. (1982). *Rape in Marriage.* New York: Macmillan.

Chapter 6

Evaluation of Domestic Abuse Intervention Programs

Melanie Shepard, PhD

From its inception, the DAIP organizers recognized the need to test their assumption that certain procedural changes by law enforcement officers, court officials, and human service providers would significantly decrease the number and severity of assaults against women. This was particularly important because they had no comprehensive model on which to base the interagency approach. Practitioners were skeptical of the claims of the women's shelter staff and the newly organized DAIP that much of the violence could be ended by changing institutional responses to batterers.

Each policy and procedure the project sought to have implemented needed to be examined against the experiences of the women they were designed to protect. The project has identified three challenges in this regard: evaluating the compliance of practitioners with interagency policies, evaluating the impact of those policies on the protection of individual women seeking help from the system, and evaluating the impact of intervention with abusers in terms of deterrence from acts of violence in current and subsequent relationships.

The project not only required major policy shifts of each participating agency but equally important, it required that each agency document for interagency review its

163

practices on each case. In 1991, the chief of the Duluth Police Department addressed a group of mental health practitioners and educators being trained to use this educational curriculum:

> I took a wait-and-see attitude on this project. I was the training officer when the shelter advocates first approached the department about experimenting with a mandatory arrest policy. Frankly, I was skeptical. I'd seen a lot of these cases in my years on patrol and I knew how ambivalent many victims were about using the courts. Our chief was about ready to retire so he agreed to a six-month experimental policy. During that time half of the officers were required to arrest when there was probable cause that the victim was assaulted and the assault caused any kind of physical injury or involved a weapon. The other officers continued to use their discretion. When the results came in a year later, I was chief and I was convinced that the policy was definitely leading to an improvement in how we handled the cases and how the rest of the system was operating. When I issued a permanent policy limiting the use of mediation and separation to those cases in which there was no injury and requiring arrest when there was injury, officers were very resistant. When our policy also included opening up dispatchers' records and arrest and investigation reports to review by a "project monitor," administrators were resistant. But in the end, all of the agencies involved had to be willing to change their practices, share information, and submit to a review of records that ensured compliance from everyone in the system.

Evaluation activities have been an important part of the development of the Domestic Abuse Intervention Project. The DAIP grew out of an experimental project that included an evaluation component. Since that time the program has been concerned both with process evaluation, to determine how the project has been implemented, and with outcome evaluation, to determine its effectiveness.

EVALUATION OF THE IMPLEMENTATION OF POLICIES

Determining how new policies and procedures are actually being implemented in a community initiating an intervention project is essential. Project staff must evaluate what is happening to cases as they progress through the system. Documentation of arrest, prosecution, and conviction rates and court orders can occur as part of the ongoing process of monitoring the criminal justice system. Examining data over time can help to identify trends which suggest that the system's response is changing. This data may also reveal problems that were not previously apparent and be used to make the case for procedure or policy changes.

The DAIP has a court monitor who examines police and dispatcher reports to assess whether or not an arrest should have been made; files reports with the police department when there are concerns about the police response in individual cases; reviews court documents to determine whether or not the prosecutor is dropping cases and if so, on what basis; monitors the court's action in criminal and civil cases; and maintains contact with judges and prosecutors to discuss concerns as they arise.

When the data suggest repeated problems in a certain area, the DAIP initiates policy changes. For example, records showed a gradual increase from 1986 to 1988 in the number of arrests of both parties. At the same time the shelter staff noted an increase in the number of women complaining that they were being arrested for defending themselves. The court monitor contacted 10 women who had been arrested over a 3-month period and interviewed them about their arrests. From their stories and a review of police reports, four of the women clearly had been acting in self-defense, and two others were very likely doing so. In four cases the women had initiated the violence and were then assaulted; these four arrests were consistent with department policy. With this information, DAIP staff met with the police chief and training officer to add language to the arrest policy that would eliminate arrests for violence used in self-defense and to schedule a round of training sessions to explain this new language. The change required officers to document how they had established probable cause that each person arrested had committed an assault and how the possibility of self-defense had been excluded. The language change and subsequent training immediately reduced the number of arrests of both partners.

It is important to learn directly from battered women what their experiences have been with community agencies. In 1984–85, the DAIP, in consultation with 11 formerly battered women, developed a questionnaire to determine the level of satisfaction with seven aspects of community intervention: initial police calls, prosecution of criminal cases, the civil court process, legal advocacy provided by the shelter, educational groups for women, probation and judicial involvement in criminal cases, and the counseling and education groups for batterers. The questionnaire was mailed to a random sample of women 2 years after their initial contact with the system. Most of the respondents reported that they had favorable experiences with the police, shelter, civil court, and groups. They reported less favorable experiences with probation officers and prosecutors.

The respondents were invited to a community forum to discuss the results of the survey and to help the DAIP and shelter staff interpret the data. As a result, 31 recommendations were made for altering procedures or policies and 42 women agreed to serve on committees formed to follow up on their implementation. Eventually, 23 of the recommendations were implemented through meetings with representatives from the criminal justice system.

EVALUATION OF THE IMPACT OF INTERVENTION

When developing an evaluation system, programs need to decide what results must be achieved for their efforts to be considered successful. Although the overall goal is to eliminate domestic abuse, various programs have developed objectives that address this problem in different ways. Some programs emphasize changing the behavior of men, whereas others are concerned with helping couples to improve their relationships. The DAIP has emphasized protecting women from domestic assault by increasing the responsiveness of the criminal justice system. This has influenced the manner in which the program has been evaluated.

The first study conducted at the DAIP focused on police intervention, as the project initially sought to change police procedures. Novak and Galaway (1983) compared cases in which police used officer discretion with cases in which police implemented a mandatory arrest policy. A 12-month follow-up interview with victims showed little difference between the two groups based solely on arrest in terms of repeated violence, although women whose assailants were court mandated to participate in the DAIP group program were less likely to have experienced renewed violence.

The project's concern with increasing the safety of battered women was also reflected in the previously discussed survey of battered women. Sixty percent of the women reported that they felt safer when the assailant was participating in education and counseling groups. Eighty percent reported that the combined response of the police, courts, DAIP, and the shelter had been helpful or very helpful in ending the abuse.

One DAIP study focused on changes in abusive behavior at different phases of the counseling and education program (Shepard, 1987). Lower rates of abuse were reported by battered women and batterers at later program phases, with significant reductions in physical and psychological abuse occurring during the first 3 months of the program. Lower rates of abuse were reported at a 1-year follow-up of battered women. Battered women consistently reported that the batterers were significantly more abusive than the batterers themselves reported.

EVALUATION OF RECIDIVISM

A more recent study examined abusive behavior over a 5-year follow-up period (Shepard, 1992). The earlier studies reviewed information obtained from battered women, whereas this study reviewed police and court records. The records provided information about assaults that had occurred in other relationships and were used to determine recidivism rates. Of the 100 men included in the sample, 40 were identified as recidivists because they had fallen into one or more recidivism categories: 22 had been convicted again for domestic assault, 15 had been the subject of orders for protection because of domestic assault, and 33 had been police suspects for domestic assault.

MEASUREMENT ISSUES

In each of these studies, decisions had to be made about how to measure abuse and from whom to collect information. Programs can collect data from batterers and battered women to determine reported rates of abusive behavior, as well as their experiences with the counseling and education program or criminal justice system. Program participants can provide staff with important qualitative information about their experiences through in-depth interviews.

Previously developed questionnaires frequently do not fit the evaluation needs of programs. The DAIP has found it necessary to design its own questionnaires in many situations. Although instruments have been developed to measure abuse, they were not found to meet the needs of the DAIP because they did not conceptualize abuse in terms of power and control issues and were not designed for both men and women respondents regarding both physical and psychological abuse. The Abusive Behavior Inventory (ABI) (Appendix 4) was developed in consultation with DAIP staff and battered women, and was based on the Power and Control Wheel used by the program. Initial research suggests that the ABI is a reliable and valid instrument (Shepard & Campbell, 1992).

Currently the DAIP is using the ABI to develop a self-administered evaluation tool for women who have been battered. This evaluation will be both an aid for decision making about the likelihood of a woman's gaining autonomy in her relationship and an educational tool to help her understand the complex nature of battering.

CONCLUSION

Program evaluation is an important part of being accountable to battered women and the community. Intervention programs must take the time to examine critically their assumptions about how the criminal justice system is responding and the impact of the intervention. Domestic abuse intervention is a relatively new field in which there must be room for innovation, evaluation, and modification to develop effective intervention strategies.

Domestic abuse programs must carefully consider the reason an evaluation is to be conducted. An evaluation carried out to demonstrate to a funding source a program's effectiveness will differ from one conducted to improve program services or to influence policy development. Depending on the need, programs may choose rigorous evaluation designs or less formal methods. Any evaluation should be discussed with program staff and, if indicated, program modifications should be considered and implemented. Evaluation efforts are rarely entirely favorable, particularly as our research suggests that many batterers are not amenable to change (Shepard, 1992). Although program goals must remain high, practitioners must also remember that they are not easily achieved.

REFERENCES

Novak, S., & Galaway, B. (1983). *Domestic abuse intervention project final report.* Unpublished manuscript.

Shepard, M. (1987, July). *Intervention with men who batter.* Paper presented at Third National Conference for Family Violence Researchers, Durham, NH.

Shepard, M. (1992, September). Predicting batterer recidivism five years after intervention. *Journal of Family Violence.* 7: 167–178.

Shepard, M., & Campbell, J. (1992, September). The abusive behavior inventory: A measure of psychological and physical abuse. *Journal of Interpersonal Violence.* 7: 291–305.

Chapter 7

Batterers' Programs, Battered Women's Movement, and Issues of Accountability

Tineke Ritmeester, PhD

The first interagency intervention programs were organized by activists in the battered women's movement in the late 1970s.* They focused on effecting changes in the way the police and courts handle individual domestic abuse cases, and they usually included a rehabilitation component as an integral part of a larger intervention strategy. These programs valued the existence of education or counseling for men as important, but viewed them as secondary to criminal justice reform work. Their focus was primarily on the institutional supports for battering and the victim-blaming practices of police, courts, and mental health agencies. Programs such as the DAIP, AMEND in Denver, and the Alternatives to Violence programs in Hawaii fall into this category.

Recognizing that a program focusing on intervention with batterers can have problems being accountable, organizers of the DAIP ensured that the planning and implementation of its program would be heavily influenced by shelter advocates, shelter residents, women in shelter educational groups, and formerly battered women working

---

* The author wishes to acknowledge the assistance of Lori Ottman in conducting the survey discussed in this chapter.

on confronting violence against women. The shelter participates in the training and selection of DAIP staff and group facilitators. The DAIP has committed itself not to compete with the shelter for funding and to meet with the shelter before advocating for any major shifts in policies, procedures, or legislation that impacts the way institutions respond to battered women and their abusers. Research and data collection procedures are divided between the shelter and the DAIP, and planned and interpreted cooperatively. These efforts are all a part of a system of accountability measures the program has taken over the years to ensure that the project maintain as its first priority the protection of women and children. Coral McDonnell, who has worked at the DAIP since it began, discusses the program's accountability to battered women:

> Every time we decide to try something new we talk it over with women who have used the system. Will this work or not? If so, how can it best work? We've had hundreds of arguments over the years about what groups should be like. Should we push for jail or not in a particular case? Is 10 days enough or 30 too many? We must eventually ask these questions against the criteria, will it make her safe and free to be herself? That gets lost sometimes.
>
> We offer groups in lieu of jail but only on the condition of no more violence. To be accountable to women means we must know what women are experiencing, be clear that the violence is his problem, not hers, and understand that her reactions are always influenced by the violence she has experienced in the past and has been threatened with in the future. For the DAIP, the bottom line is the commitment of all agencies to fulfill their moral and social obligations to abused women. Seventy-five percent of our budget goes to keeping the system informed and using its powers of intervention to ensure women's safety. Only 25% is spent on the rehabilitation of individual men.

Interagency programs such as the DAIP were preceded by programs for batterers organized by men who wanted to end violence against women. EMERGE in Boston and RAVEN (Rape and Violence End Now) in St. Louis are two of the oldest such programs that offer counseling and educational services for men who batter. Initially, these programs were met with a great deal of suspicion and sometimes outright hostility from women who were still struggling to provide shelter and food for battered women and their children. In the first efforts to organize men's programs to curtail violence against women, organizers of EMERGE and RAVEN were careful to base their analysis of battering on the experiences of battered women. The protection of women is the first intervention priority for profeminist batterers' programs.

Even though these programs devote most of their work and resources to rehabilitating and changing individual batterers, their profeminist approach obliges them to be accountable to the feminist shelter movement. From this profeminist perspective sexism is defined as "power and prejudice based on sex" (Diener, 1986, p. 7). It defines violence more broadly as "any act that causes the victim to do something she doesn't want to do, prevents her from doing something she wants to do, or causes her to be afraid" (Adams, 1988, p. 191). Physical violence need not be involved to control and dominate the victim, "since intimidating acts, such as punching walls, verbal threats, and psychological abuse can achieve the same results" (Adams, 1988, p. 191).

For RAVEN, helping batterers change or increasing sanctions on them is not enough. RAVEN encourages all men in the community to unlearn sexism—in a sense, to subvert patriarchal cultural practices.[1] Violence perpetrated by individual men against individual women is understood to be informed and licensed by a patriarchal society that renders more social power to men than to women. The profeminist materials produced by these groups have focused on the responsibility of men to confront other men on the issues of sexism and misogyny as well as on the pivotal importance of addressing institutional condoning of battering in their communities.

As batterers' programs began to spread throughout the United States in the 1980s and 1990s, it soon became apparent that there would exist very different models, not all of which have the same feminist commitment to battered women as do programs such as EMERGE, RAVEN and the DAIP (Adams, 1988, p. 192). Particular techniques may be similar, but "preferred modality, emphasis, and timing of interventions give differing messages to men about allocating responsibility for their violence and about what preconditions to non-violence (if any) are expected" (Adams, 1988, p. 196).

Most new programs now being organized are being started by mental health centers through the efforts of individual private mental health practitioners. The focus of these programs or services varies tremendously. Some work on restoring marriages and relationships by looking at violence as a manifestation of a dysfunctional relationship, whereas some work exclusively with abusers on anger management, stress reduction, and interpersonal communicating skills. Others adapt program models such as that of the DAIP. The orientation of these programs has been largely determined by the theoretical perspective of individual therapists or counselors who have put battering on the agenda of their respective agencies.[2]

Although most batterers' programs work with court-mandated clients, many of them are not part of a community interagency network and do not commit significant resources to advocate for institutional reforms. The personal ideology and backgrounds of key organizers, the availability of resources, and the connection of these programs to shelter and advocacy programs for battered women are major factors in how and to what extent these programs have come to understand their role in a community response to battering, their role in working with individual men who batter, and finally their role in working with the women who are abused by those men.

As new programs continue to form and old ones begin to reexamine the structures they have created, important decisions need to be made about the relationship of batterers' programs to the national organized battered women's movement, to the local battered women's advocacy/shelter program, and to individual battered women. Each such decision will inevitably affect the local shelter as well as the women it serves. For this reason it is critical that the concept of accountability is addressed at the very inception of these programs. The counselor must not be accountable solely to the client; the safety of the batterer's partner must supersede the confidentiality between counselor and batterer. Given that any program for batterers is situated in the same public sphere as the battered women's movement, any definition of accountability ideally should include an explicit commitment to cooperate with shelter programs.

No one expects that court intervention and rehabilitation of abusive men will stop all abuse, but it is the right of shelter/advocacy programs to expect that these endeavors will do no harm to women. In each aspect of planning an intervention program organizers must ask how their proposed practice will enhance rather than diminish women's ability to live a life free of violence. Whether the particular planners are aware of it or not, programs for batterers are situated in a political and historical context of the feminist antiviolence movement. Understanding of that movement can help those who start intervention programs work cooperatively with their local advocacy program.

BATTERED WOMEN'S MOVEMENT: A BRIEF OVERVIEW

The American suffragette movement encompassed the first modern organized resistance to violence against women. It did not organize services for women as we know them today, nor, in those pre-Freudian days, was the notion of organizing personal change groups for individual batterers even imaginable. In a sense the suffragette movement was a precursor of the contemporary domestic abuse intervention movement. Rather than focusing on the relationship between a man and the woman he batters, it too focused on institutional change and on eliminating the legal right of men to abuse their wives. Spokespersons of the suffragette movement, including Cady Stanton, supported the temperance movement because of the large number of housewives who were being mobilized to strike back at the saloons which took their husbands' paychecks, filled the men with alcohol, and sent them home at the end of a long work week broke, drunk, and violent. In fact, it could be argued that those bands of women that smashed the windows of the saloons, pulled out the men, and lobbied relentlessly for prohibition constitute the first organized battered women's groups in this country.

As legislative bodies sought to address the grievances of women without giving them political power through the vote, state after state began criminalizing wife abuse and discontinued the practice of regulating it. In 1871, Alabama and Massachusetts became the first states to criminalize all physical assaults by husbands against their wives. By the end of World War I, all states had outlawed wife beating, and the temperance laws were enacted. But police and courts in every state used their new powers of intervention selectively.

For the next 60 years wife beating continued with only isolated acts of organized resistance. Women in Chiswick, England, changed all of that in 1972 by taking over a public building and demanding that the government participate in the protection of women and children from violent husbands and fathers. Activists in the women's movements, particularly in the U.S. antirape movement, recognized the social condition of the women in Chiswick and were inspired by their courage. In just 1 year shelters began organizing in cities such as Boston, Portland (Oregon), and St. Paul, paving the way for what soon would become a national shelter movement.

As battered women across the country crowded into these buildings, their stories revealed a horrendous pattern of institutional callousness and hostility toward them. Shelter activists soon learned that a tremendous amount of work needed to be done to change the very institutions obligated to protect citizens. One of the most glaring problems was that the system's response to violence against women in their homes was to remove the women and their children rather than the abusers. Before 1976 only a handful of states provided the legal tools for arresting or removing abusers from their homes. Proposals for legislative changes allowing police to arrest batterers and family court judges to evict them met with stiff resistance. Legislation criminalizing the rape of wives, controlling forced mediation between batterers and their partners, and increasing penalties for second and third convictions of violence also met with opposition. In state after state, shelter workers organized groups of women to meet in legislative offices and testify at hearings, bringing their pictures, stories, and files for public viewing. Legislation changed and shelters were funded, though minimally. By 1986, more than 50 percent of the states had passed laws allowing women to get civil protection orders and allowing police to initiate arrests in domestic assaults.

All of these measures resulted in new questions: "What do we do with the arrested assailants? What do we do with the men excluded from their homes?" The solution of organizing rehabilitation services for abusers was a new one, one that the shelter advocates didn't have the resources to deal with. At the same time, they didn't trust the mental health practitioners who had so strongly resisted their efforts to change the accepted practices of marriage counseling and mediation as an intervention strategy. The question remained: Could batterers' programs help battered women?

IMPACT OF BATTERERS' PROGRAMS ON ADVOCACY PROGRAMS AND BATTERED WOMEN

In 1991, under the auspices of the DAIP, the author conducted an impact survey of 76 shelters for battered women in 30 states and the Province of Ontario (Canada) to determine the perspective of shelter workers on the impact of batterers' programs on their work and on battered women. The responses were mixed, with some shelters reporting that the batterer's program in their community had in many ways improved the responses of the system to battered women, the ability of shelters to work with women to stop the violence in their lives, and safety for battered women. Others reported just the opposite.

A summary follows of some of these responses interspersed with commentary from interviews with facilitators and staff at the DAIP.

Thirty-eight percent of the respondents found that the existence of a batterers' program in their community decreased the pressure on women to stay with their partners, 37% found it to remain the same, and 25% found it to increase the pressure on women. Thirty-seven percent agreed, 15% strongly, that the communication between the batterers' program and the partners of men in the program was appropriate and adequate. However, half (48%) of shelters surveyed felt the communication was either inappropriate or inadequate. Madeline Duprey, a staff member at the DAIP, elaborates on the importance of maintaining this communication.

> When I facilitate a women's orientation I'm always aware of how varied women's attitudes to the program are. Some women are really very hopeful that we can somehow get through to him in a way she hasn't been able to. Other women are guarded, thinking that we want her to help him to change. At orientation sessions we are very blunt with women about the chances of their partners changing to the point that they will be safe and free to live an autonomous life without violence, threats, or coercion. I tell women that if they are going to leave the relationship to plan to do it in the safest way and ideally to do it when we are working with him. It is also important that women and not the facilitators evaluate his change process. If women ask us, "How is he doing in the group?" or "Is he making any progress?" we ask her to answer those questions herself, based on whether or not his behavior toward her has changed. I think we are very clear that success is measured not by who stays together and who breaks up but by the degree of personal freedom women experience after using the system.

One of most common tactics abusers use to control their victims is to threaten to obtain custody of the children if she leaves him. Thirty-nine percent of the shelters surveyed indicated that the batterer's program in their community enhanced the abuser's position in visitation and custody battles, 47% found it to remain unchanged, and 14% reported a decrease. Given the power that threats of gaining custody have over battered women, these figures give rise to serious concerns about how to structure a program so it does not become a tool used against women. Again Madeline Duprey, who also coordinates the Visitation Center at the DAIP, explains.

About 3 years after the program started we noticed a big increase in court rulings in disputed custody cases favoring men who had completed our program. We suspected two things were occurring. The first was that many men in the program were starting to get "system wise" and were trying to use the police and legal system against their partners. For example, there was an increase in reports of welfare fraud made by abusers against their partners. Men who had been excluded from their homes through protection orders put pressure on their partners to drop the orders by calling case workers and reporting them for holding Tupperware parties and earning extra income through babysitting, ironing, or cutting hair.

Some men who had already been arrested once knew on second or third call how to make sure that a double arrest was made. But the most devastating tactic to women is when her batterer begins fighting for custody or joint custody and uses his participation in the DAIP as evidence that he has worked through his problems while claiming she has not.

We've taken several steps to keep ourselves from being used against battered women. The first was for group facilitators to agree that their observations of men in groups gave them no basis to make statements to the court supporting a man's request for increased visitation or custody.

Secondly, we started a visitation center, which is open three times a week, where the exchange of children can happen in a respectful manner. Both parties are able to have third-party documentation when either party fails to follow court orders regarding visitation, and men with no place to visit their children or men who were abusive to their children have a comfortable place to be with their kids.

We are now developing a protocol and procedural guide for all court and human service professionals involved in any aspect of decision making regarding custody, visitation, or termination of parental rights. Again, our efforts are to shift the focus of the system's intervention from pressuring her to somehow stop his violence to using its institutional powers to stop him.

Forty-eight percent of the respondents found that victim-blaming practices by the court had remained constant after the establishment of a batterers' program, 45% noted a decrease, and 7% indicated an increase. On the issue of the police colluding with the abuser and seeing him as the victim, 48% of the respondents indicated no change, 35% found it to have decreased, and 17% noted an increase. Again, these varied reactions demonstrate the pivotal importance of program design; it can either contribute to or reduce victim-blaming practices. One staff person at the DAIP accounts for the differences.

A batterers' program has a lot of influence in how the court defines the problem. For example, if a batterers' group is called "an anger management group" then judges, prosecutors, probation officers will all come to see the violence as an eruption of his anger. The whole idea of how he systematically defines and controls her life becomes misunderstood. If the courts don't understand that these assaults are always intentional, sometimes carefully planned, and frequently measured to elicit a certain response, they will inevitably make decisions in sentencing or revocation hearings that don't work for women. The first step to eliminate victim blaming is to eliminate language which obscures what happened.

I also think the monitoring and exchange of information that flows from police officer to advocate to prosecutor to probation officer to counselor and back through that same system is crucial to put a check on victim blaming. The more we communicate and hold our individual actions up to collective review, the less likely we are to be conned and the victim to be blamed.

Forty-seven percent of the respondents found that judges are more inclined to impose jail sentences for repeat offenders as a result of the batterers' program, 47% noted no change, and 8%, a decrease. Sixty-three percent indicated no change in police arrest of abusers, 35% noted an increase, and 2%, a decrease. Fifty-two percent found that the system is not more willing to warn victims of danger of assault, 41% saw this willingness increased, and 7% noted a decrease. Forty-eight percent indicated that prosecution of domestic assault remained the same, a significant 44% noted an increase, and 8%, a decrease. Although more than half of the shelters reported that the establishment of an abusers' program had no impact on how police and judges use their powers of punitive sanctions, many shelters found intervention projects to improve the system's protection of battered women. Tyran Schroyer, coordinator for men's groups at the DAIP, sheds light on these results:

> You can adopt all the policies in the world which are supposed to protect battered women but if the system isn't clear about what is victim blaming and what is truly helpful to a man who is battering, women are going to continue to suffer.
>
> Even though the project's been around for over 10 years, I'm surprised at some of the attitudes still around. People seem to want to blame women for being afraid. If she's too afraid to testify against him you still hear the threats to charge her or stop sending squads out to help her. Policies can and will be used against women unless there is a constant monitoring and constant sense of outrage when a woman gets punished for a man's violence.

Fifty-five percent of shelters reported a decrease in violence as a result of the batterers' program, 42% noted no change, and 4 percent saw an increase in violence. Forty-nine percent noted no change in the abuser's use of sexual violence, 40% noted a decrease, and 11%, an increase. Forty-seven percent noted no change in the safety of battered women, 42% saw an increase, and 12%, a decrease. Forty-six percent found that the abuser's use of emotional abuse remained the same, 42% noted an increase, and 12%, a decrease.

Although most shelters felt batterers' programs decreased violence against women, almost half felt they had no impact or, worse, actually increased the violence. Eighty-eight percent of the shelters responding perceived that the batterers' programs either had no impact on reducing emotional abuse or actually increased emotional abuse of women. This perception of shelters and the limited resources available to protect women explains many of the ambivalent feelings shelter activists have about batterers' programs.

CONCLUSION

During the past 15 years, programs for batterers have emerged from the profeminist men's movement, the feminist criminal justice reform movement, and the mental health field. Regardless of their different approaches, most of them share a basic interest in ensuring that they do not further endanger women. Yet according to the results of a 1991 survey of shelters, many batterers' programs do not improve the situation for battered women and a few actually make it worse. The survey leaves no doubt that shelter advocates believe programs for batterers are more effective and improve the protection of battered women when they work closely with shelter/advocacy programs. This important relationship has not been established in most communities.

An unsettling finding of the survey confirms the initial fear of shelter workers, many of whom have themselves been battered, that some batterers who go through these programs frequently shift from using physical violence to other forms of abuse to control their partners.

The experience of the DAIP and seemingly many other communities has been that victim-blaming practices and collusion with batterers are less likely to occur when battered women and shelter advocates are actively involved in the planning, implementation, monitoring, and evaluation of each aspect of the intervention process.

NOTES

1. These activities include raising money from men for rape crisis centers or battered women's shelters; doing child care for feminist events; joining the National Organization of Changing Men; support profeminist music (e.g., Geof Morgan, Romanovsky and Phillips, Fred Small); confronting sexist language and rape "jokes"; confronting sexist ads, including promotion of macho men; confronting heterosexism and homophobia; educating heterosexual men about responsibility for birth control; and subscribing to *Changing Men* magazine. Although listening to profeminist music or reading *Changing Men* alone will hardly contribute to greater accountability toward battered women, this cluster of recommended activities indicates that accountability requires a praxis that goes well beyond one-dimensional individual change.

2. There exist five clinical approaches to battering: the insight, ventilation, interaction, cognitive behavior, and profeminist models (Adams, 1988, p. 178).

REFERENCES

Adams, D. (1988). Treatment models of men who batter: A profeminist analysis. In K. Yllö & M. Bograd (Eds.), *Feminist perspectives on wife abuse*. Beverly Hills: Sage.

Diener, S. (1986, July–August). Profeminism and Nonviolence. *The Nonviolent Activist*, 7–8.

Conclusion

Ending the Violence

This book presents theory, teaching techniques, group assignments, and even a few pearls of wisdom. But all of this is mechanical. It doesn't describe the human part of teaching. The images of a men's group are missing.

The Duluth men's groups meet in an old red sandstone building that used to be a Catholic grade school. Most groups are held in the evening. Smoking is not allowed in the building so the early arrivals stand on the front step under a life-size statue of Jesus, smoking until the group begins. At exactly 7 p.m., they flick their cigarettes out into the parking lot and file into the classroom.

Some of the men wear hats. The baseball type dominates in style, and each advertises something different: a bait and tackle shop, a favorite beer, a lumber yard, or a hockey team.

Some of the men sit next to a friend in the group and exchange a few words as the room fills. Others sit off as far as possible in the corner, knowing that their self-imposed isolation will be quickly ended because each group starts by moving the chairs into a close circle.

The two facilitators are up front getting video equipment and handouts ready and cleaning off the blackboard. A couple of the men greet them with a quip, a nod, or a single-fingered half-salute. Others just move in and take a seat.

About half the men take off their jackets; half don't. No one takes off his hat. Some of the men wear suits; most wear blue jeans.

One of the facilitators says, "OK, let's move the chairs in." The group has started. What comes next is the part we can't teach. It's the human part of this process that each of us doing this work has brought to the room.

This work begins with commitment. It begins with a commitment to women who are called names, beaten, kicked, pushed, stabbed, held hostage, raped, and subjected to constant attack on their very essence as human beings. It begins with a commitment to these men, too—not to the part of them that unfairly uses another person, but to the part in all of us that is capable of giving and receiving love. Our work must be personal. It must involve a commitment to join with the men in refusing to participate in a system that dehumanizes all of us.

This work offers each of us the opportunity to examine some of our most basic beliefs about who we are in relationship to our partners, our friends, and our community.

Our culture and our society encourage us to see power as the ability to control. The extent to which one is able to influence events, to acquire and control increasing amounts of resources, and to influence the behavior and actions of others is the measure of his or her power. Both the facilitator and the men in the group share in that cultural perspective.

To move from a society in which individuals seek power, and its corresponding ability to control, to a society in which its members seek collective and personal empowerment and its creative power is a complex process.

Any system that gives one group power over another group dehumanizes both those with too much power and those without enough power. But what is the role of the individual batterer in the overall scheme of things? If we see him as only a victim of a larger system in which he has no say and is merely a pawn of a sexist society, we take away his individual responsibility, making it less likely that he will change.

This program in all its aspects rejects the notion of men as victims of sexism. Ultimately, each of us must be held accountable for the choices we make. The use of this curriculum challenges men to see their use of violence as a choice—not an uncontrolled reaction to their past, their anger, or their lack of skills—but a choice.

The socialization of men and women in this society teaches us to adhere to strictly defined roles that in the end separate us from each other. This curriculum challenges much of what the men believe, and in the process challenges those of us who teach it.

The work we do with men's groups can extend far beyond the limited concepts we are able to discuss in this book. The exploration of values and beliefs can bring facilitators to a deeper understanding of their own values regarding power, children, winning and losing, sexuality, and intimacy.

Throughout these pages are the voices of men. Hundreds of hours of men's meetings are on tape. The short segments we use in the text of the book illustrate specific points but leave the spirit of the groups back in the classroom. They don't show the times humorous things happen, the times the group loses focus and goes nowhere, the times the men really help each other out, the times the men are vulnerable, or the times the men who are leaving talk about their experiences and say goodbye.

Many men in these groups will stop physically and sexually abusing women but many won't. It is crucial that those of us who have some influence in how the community responds to those who continue to batter their partners know the difference between compassion and collusion. No man is helped by our collusion, no woman is hurt by our compassion. A facilitator must recognize that sometimes the most compassionate thing we can do for a man who batters is to physically prevent him from being violent. Jail, exclusion orders, and the denial of visitation are often needed to stop his violence. Using them does not mean the groups have failed, but that that man has not yet made the decision to change.

We encourage each man and each woman who takes on the task of facilitating groups for men who batter to walk into the room mindful of the women whose lives have been diminished by the violence of those you seek to help. If the group was encircled by those women, what jokes, what conversations, what expectations, and what explanations would seem appropriate?

This curriculum can lead to true empowerment in men. It challenges men to take the risk to stop controlling, to stop having all the power. It asks men to give women the choice to love them. It asks them to respect women, to give up the privileged status our society has given them. The curriculum gives each of the men the choice to be in an equal relationship with a woman, which means that he will feel pain, will sometimes lose and won't always get to decide. Making that choice allows him to be fully human.

APPENDICES

All of the following materials may be duplicated.

Power and Control Wheel

VIOLENCE

PHYSICAL · SEXUAL

USING COERCION AND THREATS
Making and/or carrying out threats to do something to hurt her • threatening to leave her, to commit suicide, to report her to welfare • making her drop charges • making her do illegal things.

USING INTIMIDATION
Making her afraid by using looks, actions, gestures • smashing things • destroying her property • abusing pets • displaying weapons.

USING ECONOMIC ABUSE
Preventing her from getting or keeping a job • making her ask for money • giving her an allowance • taking her money • not letting her know about or have access to family income.

USING EMOTIONAL ABUSE
Putting her down • making her feel bad about herself • calling her names • making her think she's crazy • playing mind games • humiliating her • making her feel guilty.

POWER AND CONTROL

USING MALE PRIVILEGE
Treating her like a servant • making all the big decisions • acting like the "master of the castle" • being the one to define men's and women's roles

USING ISOLATION
Controlling what she does, who she sees and talks to, what she reads, where she goes • limiting her outside involvement • using jealousy to justify actions.

USING CHILDREN
Making her feel guilty about the children • using the children to relay messages • using visitation to harass her • threatening to take the children away.

MINIMIZING, DENYING AND BLAMING
Making light of the abuse and not taking her concerns about it seriously • saying the abuse didn't happen • shifting responsibility for abusive behavior • saying she caused it.

PHYSICAL · SEXUAL

VIOLENCE

Equality Wheel

NONVIOLENCE

NEGOTIATION AND FAIRNESS

Seeking mutually satisfying resolutions to conflict • accepting change • being willing to compromise.

NON-THREATENING BEHAVIOR

Talking and acting so that she feels safe and comfortable expressing herself and doing things.

ECONOMIC PARTNERSHIP

Making money decisions together • making sure both partners benefit from financial arrangements.

RESPECT

Listening to her non-judgmentally • being emotionally affirming and understanding • valuing opinions.

EQUALITY

SHARED RESPONSIBILITY

Mutually agreeing on a fair distribution of work • making family decisions together.

TRUST AND SUPPORT

Supporting her goals in life • respecting her right to her own feelings, friends, activities and opinions.

RESPONSIBLE PARENTING

Sharing parental responsibilities • being a positive non-violent role model for the children.

HONESTY AND ACCOUNTABILITY

Accepting responsibility for self • acknowledging past use of violence • admitting being wrong • communicating openly and truthfully.

NONVIOLENCE

DOMESTIC ABUSE INTERVENTION PROJECT (DAIP)

CONTRACT FOR PARTICIPATION

_____ court pending
_____ volunteered

Name _____ On _____ I _____ was court ordered

to participte in the DAIP counseling/education program.

1.___ I agree to attend an orientation session at the Damiano Center, 206 West Fourth Street, Room _____ on (day/date) _____ (time) _____. I understand that I cannot miss the orientation session without making prior arrangments.

2.___ I agree to attend _____ counseling sessions at _____, _____
Groups meet (day/time) _____. I agree to contact my counselor _____
by _____ to make an appointment to start the group. Phone _____ .
___ I agree to attend _____ educational groups at _____ to begin _____
at (time) _____ on (day) _____. Facilitators _____.
___ Other _____

(I understand that I may be charged a fee for service.)

3.___ I understand that I cannot miss more than two (2) sessions during the first 14 week phase and no more than two (2) sessions during the second 12 week phase. I understand that I must contact my counselor or the DAIP if I will be absent and agree to make up any session missed. Failure to comply will result in suspension and, if court ordered, referral back to the court.

4.___ If recommended I agree to obtain a chemical dependency evaluation and follow any recommendations.

5.___ I understand that by Civil Protection I am excluded from the Petitioner's residence.
___ I understand that no one, including the Petitioner, _____, can change the Civil Protection Order without the permission of the court. I understand that I may ask the court for a review hearing to request changes in the order.

6.___ I understand my counselors/facilitators will report my attendance, any acts of violence and an evaluation of my progress to the DAIP.

7.___ I understand the DAIP will report information regarding my partipation in the program or reported acts of violence to the court.

8.___ I understand that the DAIP will contact (victim) _____ to obtain a history of abuse. They will provide her/him with the name of my counselor. She/he will also be informed of my attendance, any pending court hearings, and suspension or termination of my involvement with the DAIP.

9.___ I understand that if I move, I must notify the DAIP of change of address and telephone number.

10.___ I understand that violations of Conditions of Probation or Civil Protection Orders are grounds for removal from group and referral back to court.

11.___ I understand that I must notify the DAIP of any further police contact, service of a protection order, or any new or pending charges.

12.___ **I AGREE NOT TO BE VIOLENT WITH ANY PERSON DURING MY PARTICIPATION IN THE DAIP PROGRAM.**

I HAVE READ THIS CONTRACT AND UNDERSTAND MY REQUIREMENTS WITH THE DAIP. VIOLATION OF THE CIVIL PROTECTION ORDER MAY RESULT IN IMPRISONMENT OF UP TO NINETY (90) DAYS AND/OR A FINE OF UP TO $700. VIOLATION OF CONDITIONS OF PROBATION MAY RESULT IN REVOCATION OR PROBATION AND THE IMPOSITION OF THE ORIGINAL SENTENCE.

Participant _____ Witness _____

Date _____ 1/92

APPENDIX 4

Abusive Behavior Inventory

Here is a list of behaviors that many women report have been used by their partners or former partners. We would like you to estimate how often these behaviors occurred during the 6 months before your partner began this program. Your answers are strictly confidential.

Circle a number from the list below for each item to show your closest estimate of how often the behavior happened in your relationship with your partner or former partner during the *6 months before* he started the program.

1 = Never
2 = Rarely
3 = Occasionally
4 = Frequently
5 = Very frequently

1. Called you names and/or criticized you	1	2	3	4	5
2. Tried to keep you from doing something you wanted to do (e.g., said you couldn't go out with friends or go to a meeting).	1	2	3	4	5
3. Gave you angry stares or looks.	1	2	3	4	5
4. Prevented you from having money for your own use.	1	2	3	4	5
5. Ended a discussion with you and made the decision himself.	1	2	3	4	5
6. Threatened to hit or throw something at you.	1	2	3	4	5
7. Pushed, grabbed or shoved you.	1	2	3	4	5
8. Put down your family and friends.	1	2	3	4	5
9. Accused you of paying too much attention to someone or something else.	1	2	3	4	5
10. Put you on an allowance.	1	2	3	4	5
11. Used your children to threaten you (e.g., told you that you would lose custody or said he would leave town with the children).	1	2	3	4	5

12. Became very upset with you because dinner, housework or laundry was not ready when he wanted it or done the way he thought it should be.   1   2   3   4   5

13. Said things to scare you (e.g., told you something "bad" would happen or threatened to commit suicide).   1   2   3   4   5

14. Slapped, hit or punched you.   1   2   3   4   5

15. Made you do something humiliating or degrading (e.g., made you beg for forgiveness or ask his permission to use the car or do something).   1   2   3   4   5

16. Checked up on you (e.g., listened to your phone calls, checked the mileage on your car, or called you repeatedly at work).   1   2   3   4   5

17. Drove recklessly when you were in the car.   1   2   3   4   5

18. Pressured you to have sex in a way that you didn't like or want.   1   2   3   4   5

19. Refused to do housework or child care.   1   2   3   4   5

20. Threatened you with a knife, gun, or other weapon.   1   2   3   4   5

21. Spanked you.   1   2   3   4   5

22. Told you that you were a bad parent.   1   2   3   4   5

23. Stopped you or tried to stop you from going to work or school.   1   2   3   4   5

24. Threw, hit, kicked, or smashed something.   1   2   3   4   5

25. Kicked you.   1   2   3   4   5

26. Physically forced you to have sex.   1   2   3   4   5

27. Threw you around.   1   2   3   4   5

28. Physically attacked the sexual parts of your body.   1   2   3   4   5

29. Choked or strangled you.   1   2   3   4   5

30. Used a knife, gun, or other weapon against you.   1   2   3   4   5

APPENDIX 5

Action Plan

Name _____

Changes I am making	Specific steps

APPENDIX 6

CONTROL LOG

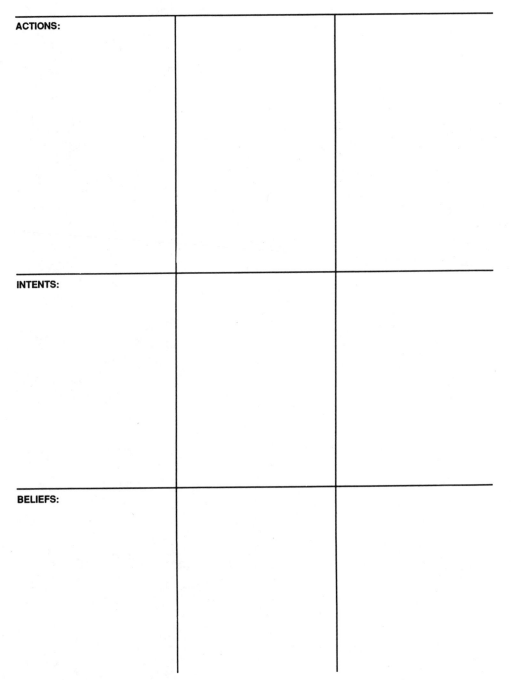

ACTIONS:

INTENTS:

BELIEFS:

INDEX